Praise for J. Keith McMullin's *Missing Mary*

A heartfelt depiction of one family's journey through Alzheimer's disease, filled with many p͟r͟ s to make things better.

The ͟ uthor of r of the Division of (͟chiatry ͟ ͟chool of Medicine

Miss Mary nearly charmed herself out of Alzheimer's, or as Keith McMullin says, Oldzheimerz. Near the end, he asks: "How much of life turns on a whisper, such as 'I love you' or 'Good-bye?'" I typed and printed this sentence. It sits on my desk as a poignant reminder to pay attention to the ones I love.

Rosemary Rawlins, author *of Learning by Accident: A Caregiver's True Story of Fear, Family, and Hope*

Alzheimer's is a devastating disease and one I know first-hand as a nurse and daughter. Between the tears and laughs, *Missing Mary* achieves the right balance to help caregivers and loved ones deal with their newfound reality.

Francine Barr, DNP, RN, NEA-BC, CEO of St. Mary's Hospital, Bon Secours Health System

As only a Southern storyteller could do, McMullin masterfully combines the heartbreak of Alzheimer's disease with laugh-out-loud entertainment and practical insights. *Missing Mary* is a must-read for caregivers.

Tom Edwards, designer for Spotify

Missing Mary is a must read for everyone. It should not be limited to only medical and nursing professionals.

Ken White, PhD, Associate Dean, University of Virginia School of Nursing

…all I ask is a merry yarn from a laughing fellow-rover,
And quiet sleep and a sweet dream when the long trick's over.

—"Sea Fever" by John Masefield

Part of proceeds to support hospice for dementia patients and their families, including the construction of Family Counseling Rooms at Bon Secours Health System.

Cover Design by Jeff Bland
Interior Design by Pamela Morrell
Editing by Erica Orloff

ISBN: 978-0-9977478-3-6

Published by

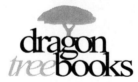

1620 SW 5th Avenue
Pompano Beach, Florida 33060
(954)788-4775
editors@editingforauthors.com
dragontreebooks.com

Missing Mary

By J. Keith McMullin

Acknowledgements

The son of a mathematician mom, I was raised to effort-lessly solve "word problems." Any pencil and the back of a cocktail napkin were all you needed. So as an adult, I had no real fear of the motherlode of all word problems—writing a book. Now that was a problem. And it got compounded because I believed Michael Pollan, the *New York Times* health reporter, who said that "Everyone has at least one story within them." Mine wasn't a story that flowed out or that needed to be pulled out or even coaxed out. Rather, it was a story that was vomited out of me. Something that had to come out with startling velocity and covered the back of the napkin.

And I believed Elie Wiesel, the holocaust survivor and human rights activist, when he said that "God created man because he loves stories."

And I believed my daughter Charlotte, when at age five sitting at the dinner table she pronounced for our family that "We speak the truth!" I will always believe in her, my happy-warrior daughter.

As if fifteen years of caregiving for my mother, father, and Great Aunt Clara was not enough work, I took the first step of this crazy writing journey late one evening at the office. That day, I had lunch with my hilarious advertising friend, Terry Taylor, at a table below a painting of Willie Nelson on blue velvet. We got a good laugh out of Velvet Willie, and he directed me to write my "first story about

Oldzheimerz before you leave the office tonight." I believed him and picked up a pen.

So with the encouragement of colleagues, friends, relatives, agents, consultants, writers, my mother-in-law Martha Wayt, and our loyal family friend and health care professional Norma Geddes, I wrote for an hour every night for a year. Thank you to the many hands that helped write this story about the many hands that helped take care of Miss Mary. With your help, I told the story the best I could and pushed print. After which, I was accepted into a James River Writers editing class taught by Erica Orloff at my church, Saint Stephen's, and the real work began. She patiently explained to me that I was writing "narrative nonfiction." It was a term that I had not heard before. Erica agreed to edit the book not once, not twice, but three times based on the problem that I had no idea what I was doing. She believed in Miss Mary, and I believed in her skill as an editor, storyteller, and senior caregiver.

And so a narrative nonfiction book about Alzheimer's dementia was born. This book would not have come to be without a do-right woman named Betty (a.k.a. Miss Mary) McMullin who raised me and a do-right woman named Martha Wayt McMullin who married me. Thank you, Marty, for believing in the story within me.

J. Keith McMullin
Gwynn's Island
Mathews, Virginia
May 27, 2015

Introduction

Mary McMullin—Miss Mary to her fans—was a do-right woman, brilliant mathematician, champion athlete, member of America's Greatest Generation and the hand behind the best Christmas cookies ever. She may have been a force of energy and one of the first women faculty at the University of Richmond in the 1960s and '70s, but she was a caregiver first, not only to her three children, but also to elderly neighbors and friends, her aunt, my aging father, our pet gerbil and assorted dogs. And me—her lucky middle son. With the spirit of a champion, Miss Mary lived life gracefully, even as Alzheimer's dementia tracked her down, took hold, and refused to let go.

Extending a hand to help her navigate the dark path of this cruel disease was my most difficult—and most worthwhile—journey in life. The injustice and pain of a slow-motion death were a given, but somehow, we experienced humor and peace on this crazy trip. As a health care executive in disease prevention and population health, I had spent years behind a desk evaluating chronic conditions, developing and launching programs to help people improve their health and feel better. Helping my mother took me from my office overlooking the city of Richmond, Virginia, to the trenches of caregiving, sorting pills, paying bills, getting Medicare on the phone, and doing whatever possible to ease the painful loss of personhood.

Alzheimer's diminished Miss Mary's memory. Remembering her and telling the story of her remarkable spirit is a small act of resistance against her cruel tyrant. Miss Mary died on January 24, 2013 at age eighty-four. She was not motivated by money or popular fame. But she did care about helping people. I hope this story helps other caregivers navigate the dark, winding path called Alzheimer's dementia.

For years, my day job was leading a team at Health Management Corporation, a division of one of the largest health care companies in the world. In addition, I participate in a clinical program providing care for patients with dementia and delirium. The root cause of Alzheimer's dementia may not yet be clear to scientists, but some issues are painfully clear with providing care to the escalating number of seniors with dementia. For instance, when a person no longer has the mental capacity to follow the sequential steps of a care plan, who manages his or her care? When Miss Mary's doctor prescribed two powerful drugs to potentially slow the progression of Alzheimer's disease, who was going to assist her so that she remembered which pill to take after breakfast and which pill to take after dinner? And then another pill was added to the cocktail for dementia-related vertigo to help prevent dizziness and falling. If she forgot to take that pill, who was responsible for picking her up from the floor?

By way of another example, Ann was a patient in her eighties with progressing dementia who had been admitted to the Emergency Room with an acute-care need. She had been a reading specialist for elementary and middle school students with learning differences. Now in her hospital room, Ann struggled to read a newspaper story as she could not recall names or follow the storyline. She wasn't able to process new information or understand the steps outlined in her care plan. She was confused, agitated, and struggling to find words as her dementia became more severe. Her devoted husband was several years older, and his health was declining. A cab brought him to the hospital from their well-appointed assisted living facility. However, Ann did not get approval to return with him to the facility after discharge from the hospital. Her care needs for dementia had changed and surpassed what they were capable of providing. Ann was now both crazy and homeless.

Ernest was in his early nineties and while in the hospital for a procedure, he was experiencing delirium, or acute mental failure. The grandson of enslaved Africans and once a successful machinist, Ernie had outlived his wife. His kids and grandchildren were busy with successful technology careers of their own on the West Coast. For physical rehabilitation and help with his medication schedule, the caseworker had arranged for him to be admitted to a local rehab facility. In order to transfer him from the hospital to rehab, he needed pants. But no one was answering the nurse's phone calls to bring him a pair of pants, delaying discharge. Eventually, a crumpled brown paper bag appeared at the foot of his bed. In it was a pair of khakis, but they were neither his pants nor his size, ensuring a humiliating nearly-naked exit from his hospital room.

The everyday reality is that there are millions of Marys, Anns, and Ernies. More than five million in the United States and twenty-five million worldwide are suffering from Alzheimer's dementia. And Alzheimer's is just one type of dementia. In the United States alone, it is estimated that there are more than fifteen million caregivers for people with Alzheimer's disease, and Centers for Medicare & Medicaid Services (CMS) reports the annual cost of providing health care for Alzheimer's at a staggering $306,000,000,000. With an epidemic of this magnitude, caregiving seems to be taking on as many different forms as there are forms of dementia. Research paints a picture of who is likely to provide care by demographic profile[*]:

- African-American: family grouping
- Asian: oldest son
- Caucasian: spouse
- Hispanic: oldest daughter

For me, as I started my Toyota Highlander on Saturday morning to head to Miss Mary's house to manage Bills & Pills, I knew that I was not the oldest son, not the spouse, not a family grouping, and definitely not the daughter. Nonetheless, my middle son hands seemed to do just fine loading this week's pills into the plastic blue pill boxes. If you are holding this book in your hands, those hands can help get the job done, too. Alzheimer's provides the perfect training ground for us unlikely novice caregivers... when you make a mistake, your mom won't remember a thing.

Make mine a double, Pussycat.

—Miss Mary after failing a test for the first time in life,
   the driving test for seniors

[*] Myron F. Weiner, M.D., and Anne M. Lipton, M.D., Ph.D., eds. *Textbook of Alzheimer Disease and Other Dementias.* Arlington, VA: American Psychiatric Publishing, 2009, 353–366.

1
Calling Dr. Bombay

I remember lying in bed late at night in plaid boxer shorts, barely under a sheet, listening to the air conditioner wheeze trying to keep up with the stifling July heat on Gwynn's Island. With a pleasant bourbon haze, compliments of Maker's Mark, all seemed right in the world. Even the sand that made its way into the bed was more like an old childhood friend rather than anything irritating. My wife, Marty, slept next to me, her dark hair spilled across the pillow. I heard my nine-year-old daughter, Charlotte, and her friend from school in the downstairs bunk room talking, the room jam packed with words. James, my seven year old, and his buddy occupied bunk beds across the hall, unbelievably still cutting up and laughing at their competing fart sounds. Timeless humor.

My wife and I went to bed too late and too tired to bother closing blinds. Through the window, I watched the moon dance on the choppy water of Hill's Bay as it converged with the Piankatank River and Chesapeake Bay. Richard Moore and his family had invited us to their house on Cherry Point for the weekend. Off the coast of Virginia, Gwynn's Island is comfortably rundown without time-share condos or chain restaurants. It was all familiar to me. As a kid, I spent part of every summer on a deserted stretch of Virginia Beach just south of the island. With no television, air conditioning, or digital anything, we fished and crabbed, rode waves and bikes, and played another round of the game called LIFE.

Last to fall asleep, I woke first. Roosters declared it a workday. Without making noise, I slipped out of bed and pulled on cut-off shorts lying on the floor. I headed to the dock with Richard to fish for a while. We caught a couple spot but nothing big enough to clean and cook. A water-color sunrise of red and orange irked me without my first cup of coffee.

When the sun was reasonably high and it was OK to make some noise in the house, we set aside the fishing poles and headed to the kitchen. Rich made a pot of coffee, and, with addiction satisfied, we fried bacon, scrambled cheesy eggs, sliced cantaloupe and opened a box of donuts. The smell of bacon proved more than the kids could sleep through. They stumbled into the kitchen rubbing bleary eyes and passed over the melon to grab sugar-coated and deep-fried Krispy Kreme donuts. As she ate a piece of bacon, Charlotte patted my arm, "Nice try, Pops. Not as good as Grammy Mary's, but thanks for trying." I laughed hard at the jab, knowing full well she was right. I would never compete against my mom in a cook-off, no matter her advancing age. Donuts inhaled, the kids made their way outside to ride bikes, swim and kayak for another carefree summer day of big fun.

Eventually, Sunday evening came. Like the tide, the oncoming workweek pulled me back in, and I packed the sea-foam green Highlander to return to civilization. We said our goodbyes and began the journey home, crossing the bridge to Interstate 64 and heading west to Richmond, Virginia. We looked like a Norman Rockwell painting with blue-eyed and sunburned kids piled in the backseat. I drove the two hours home, pulled into our driveway in Spottswood Park, said hello to Abner the barking beagle, unpacked the car and carried a worn-out James to bed. Sweet dreams.

As I wearily headed downstairs, the telephone rang. Looking at the number on caller ID, it was not one I recognized. I was happy to ignore it.

"Keith, it might be Mary," reasoned my wife since we usually check-in on Saturdays.

A decision hung in the balance. *Do I answer the call now? Or could I put it on hold until morning? Surely my mom and ninety-seven year-old Great Aunt Clara had hit the hay.* I headed to the basement and turned on the TV to catch up on the national news, Sports Center.

"Keith, I think your mom left a message."

"Mmm-hmmm."

At the commercial, I headed back upstairs to the bathroom. As I passed the phone, the red light had that annoying blink of urgency. I ignored it. On the return trip, I paused. *Why the unusual phone number?* Still hesitating, I reached out my hand and pressed play.

"Darlin', I'm in the hospital." Click.

It was a bona fide oh-shit moment. No sweet Southern accent could soften the impact of that statement. Those five words spoken to a machine would soon change my family forever. In my Norman Rockwell picture-perfect all-American life, the fruit basket on our dinner table just got overturned. Grapes, apples and bananas spilled chaotically off the canvas.

I called her cell phone. It wasn't on. I tried the number on the machine, but got no answer. Within five miles of her house were two hospitals. Which one? Miss Mary used to take my father to St. Mary's. Marty stayed with the kids, and I drove straight to the emergency room and rushed between the sliding glass doors. All the seats in the waiting room were taken, but none by my seventy-nine year-old mother. The nun at the admissions desk checked the records: no Mary McMullin was admitted to the hospital. I had guessed wrong. Time to try E.R. door number two.

I sped to Henrico Doctor's Hospital. Anxiously, I asked the admissions nurse if Mary McMullin had been admitted. She huffed, "Yes, Mr. McMullin. The doctor has been waiting for you. Room three." I detected an eye roll. Clearly, we had a situation.

The automatic doors opened to the E.R., and I walked back. Upon entering, I felt the all-too-familiar feeling of anxiety. How many times had I been here before with my father for a cardiac event? The smell and sound of vomit splattering was not helping matters. More retching. The temperature was chilly and felt freezing cold against sunburned legs in cut-off shorts. I folded my arms and rubbed them to stay warm, sending sand to the tile floor. The woman in the centralized nurse station stood and inquired, "Are you Mr. MacMillan?"

"Yes." It was not a good time to correct her mispronunciation of my family name. A medical mob formed: several nurses, a medical technician and a very short, very angry doctor with a black uni-brow above his eyeglasses that caught stray pieces of white dandruff. This was not looking good. "How is my mother?" I stammered.

"Are you aware that your mother is showing signs of dementia and vertigo?"

"Yes, she calls them 'spells.'"

"How often does she have one of her 'spells'?"

"Occasionally, maybe once every couple of months. Usually she just lies down and rests for a while."

"Does she live alone?"

"No."

"She lives with you?"

"No, she lives with Aunt Clara."

"Her sister?"

"Her aunt."

"Her aunt? How old, exactly, is her aunt?

"Ninety-seven."

"Are you telling me that your mother is a caregiver?"

"Well, not like she was with my father. Aunt Clara is pretty self-sufficient. My mom does a lot of cooking, though."

"Excuse me? Let me explain what we know, Mr. McMullin. Your mother has a hernia. On the Wong-Baker rating scale of pain, an eight or nine out of ten. In her pain, coupled with dementia and vertigo, she fell and hit her head. She got up, probably with your ninety-seven-year-old aunt's help. Instead of calling an ambulance, she apparently changed clothes, put on make-up and *drove herself to the E.R.!*"

Dr. Scream was red-faced and determined to make his point. I was hoping for someone more along the lines of good-humored Dr. Bombay—emergency, emergency come right away with a wriggle of Samantha's lips. But this was not a thirty-minute episode of *Bewitched*. Scowling Dr. Scream continued, "With dementia-related vertigo, your mother cannot care for a ninety-seven-year-old aunt. She cannot admit herself to the E.R. And she *cannot be driving!*"

At this point in the freezing E.R., Miss Mary appeared in the doorway, barefoot and in a hospital gown. Although she was in a mess of trouble and pain with a ruptured abdominal hernia, she appeared unruffled and good-looking. "Please excuse me, Doctor, but I took all the back roads."

Dr. Scream totally lost it with us. "*I'm reporting both of you to the administrator in charge!*" The jury of nurses and technicians hammered away at me with more questions. They deliberately pointed out another family in the E.R. whose members were in shock because of a fatal car accident as they continued to cross-examine me like I was on trial for pre-meditated murder, including intent to kill my kind-hearted mother. In the barrage, they informed me they were running more tests. She was scheduled for surgery at 6:00 a.m. Norman Rockwell never painted this scene.

At 4:00 a.m. we arrived at our room, Miss Mary sleeping soundly. I answered another round of redundant questions from another person in green scrubs, and fell asleep, cold to the bone with sunburned and sandy legs sticking to the blue vinyl hospital chair. An hour later a new nurse woke us to begin prepping mom for surgery. While taking her pulse, she recognized Miss Mary as her mother-in-law's trusted golf partner. She leaned over and hugged her, and the two began talking about Mary's very favorite subject—grandchildren. The doctor attempted to interrupt and repeated to me that she was in excruciating pain. Just before surgery, though, she and the nurse were still chatting about the face cream my mom used to maintain flawless skin. In classic Miss Mary style, the nurse was now our very best friend and pledged to do anything to help us until the end of time.

This included talking on the phone to relatives asking about my mom's health. Hearing from the nurse was a far better solution than my older brother debating with me by phone about what was taking place directly in front of me. Miss Mary explained to her new friend with a wink, "We have lots of out-of-town experts. But the truth of the matter is, Clara and I do just fine. My son gives us a hand when we need it." As she was wheeled to the operating room, Miss Mary took off her opal and diamond ring, a heart-felt gift left to her from Aunt Betty. She slipped it to me with whispered directions, "Sugar, please keep this safe in your pocket." Good thinking. *And please explain to me, Doctor, where exactly does my mother fall on the Wong-Baker rating scale for crazy?*

Within an hour, hospital staff rolled Miss Mary back from surgery. The doctor reported the hernia operation successful. However, an MRI indicated that my mother had dementia, likely Alzheimer's. Was there a family history?

"Yes, her mother, Jewel; her grandfather, Caloway; her aunt; her sister, Sarah…"

The doctor interrupted, "Who is her primary care physician? He should be aware of these test results."

"Thank you. She has seen Dr. Gergoudis for many years."

"Your mother can't do any better than Richard Gergoudis. He will want to see these test results."

Miss Mary woke up groggy, her eyes only half open. Nonetheless, she wanted to watch women's tennis played on the grass courts at Wimbledon. Venus Williams, ranked fourteen, played Lindsay Davenport, ranked number one, for the women's title. While watching the three-hour epic battle, my mind wandered to all the things that I was not getting done. I was not checking any item off the list of yard work and office work. I was watching sports on TV and not watching Charlotte's and James's live soccer matches. My sister was not answering her phone, and clearly she was not available to help. I sat back in the recliner and got comfortable. Unbelievably, Venus kept breaking back and fighting the odds stacked against her to win the final set of the match 9-7. Miss Mary's eyes were closed and her breathing slow. For the first time in life, she looked exhausted and frail. I knew that she was not going to be breaking back and recovering quickly. And Mary would no longer be able to take care of ninety-seven-year-old Aunt Clara who was now home alone. It seemed I was the proud new owner of a senior center. I knew one thing for certain, with Alzheimer's we would not be moving forward in a straight line from point A to point B with powerful purpose like Venus on the grass court. This very odd dance with dementia would progress in a swirling, chaotic, unfamiliar motion.

* * *

While sitting in the blue vinyl chair in the hospital room, I thought about Dr. Scream making his point in the E.R. He was right. Miss Mary's spells were a growing cause for concern and had advanced beyond, "Hoo, I feel woozy." She was in need of more treatment than an Old Fashioned on the rocks, two aspirin and a nap. On my laptop, I entered "Alzheimer's disease" into Google and clicked "I'm Feeling Lucky." The Alzheimer's Association website appeared. "Alzheimer's is the sixth-leading cause of death." Lucky me. I tried a general Google Search, and more than 20,000,000 entries were listed. Sitting with a sleeping Miss Mary in her hospital room, I had plenty of time for reading. Information gathering had begun.

I had worked in health care for a long time and had easy access to subject matter experts. In the upcoming weeks and months, I talked with my colleagues who worked with conditions like dementia and delirium. Later that summer, I went kayaking with my buddy, Dr. Dave, who had a M.D. and Ph.D. in neurology. He gave me the download on Alzheimer's disease. At his suggestion, I ordered the dementia caregiver's Bible titled *The 36-Hour Day* written by Peter V. Rabins, M.D., M.P.H. and medical professionals from Johns Hopkins University and began studying. Most importantly, I started talking to my mom's primary care physician.

The truth about Alzheimer's dementia is that a caregiver can send a loved one's MRI test results to the best doctor on Earth, but he cannot cure the patient or prevent the disease.

There is no overcoming Alzheimer's; it has a one hundred percent mortality rate. Even if the person is as strong and as smart and as determined as Venus Williams, this opponent always wins and reduces you to zero.

Alzheimer's disease has been around by name for more than a century and remains a Goliath that cannot be slain, a cruel and elusive enemy. More men and women have died at the hands of Alzheimer's dementia than all the casualties combined from The Revolutionary War, The Civil War, World War I, and World War II. Clinically, it is not possible to diagnose the disease with complete accuracy until after death and an autopsy of the brain is performed. Brain tissue must be removed from inside the skull and examined under a microscope by a scientist in order to determine the exact cause of death. And even then, doctors who are expert at taking care of the sick—the second-oldest occupation in the world—can say exactly one thing with certainty about the dead patient: "Yes, she lost her mind."

When you are the one with Alzheimer's, the brain is the organ that fails you in a cell-by-cell death. Billions of cells that make up your mind slowly deteriorate until they can no longer tell your throat to swallow. Because of the complexity of the brain, Alzheimer's disease acts as a shape-shifter with as many variations as it has victims. More often than not, it first impacts the middle section of the brain, the area that generates personality, memory and emotion. In the process of dying from Alzheimer's, you lose parts of yourself and what makes you uniquely you. What you become is dependent on others for full care. You require help eating, bathing, dressing, toileting, walking. For those who care for you and love you, it is a long farewell with countless tears shed over countless days until the final goodbye. Florence, the African-American housekeeper who helped raise me, had a saying, "You've got plenty of time to lick all the pots clean in

Sorrow's kitchen." And with my new job as chief pot licker, I learned she was exactly right.

In America, our preferred solution to a health problem is a new pill. The average senior over the age of eighty is prescribed eighteen medications a year. Just say "yes" to drugs. For Alzheimer's dementia, a handful of drugs, like Aricept, try to slow to a trickle the process of losing your mind. They come with side effects, however, and add new problems that change the equation. And when you have dementia, how do you remember to take your medications for memory loss? How do you remember where you left the pillbox? How do you recall that today is Thursday and that "T" marks the compartment for Thursday's pills? Or is that "T" for Tuesday? Or is it "TH" for Thursday? Or "T" for Today? How do you remember if you have taken this morning's three pills or yesterday evening's two pills? And do you recall why you are taking these pills in the first place? What does medication adherence look like after you leave the doctor's office, drive away from Westbury Pharmacy with Medicare and Uncle Sam generously picking up the bill? The great hope to beating Alzheimer's disease is the development of a new magic pill, a blockbuster drug. But will you remember to take it? In short, Alzheimer's creates questions and problems and chaos. It is not in the business of answers or solutions or clarity. Welcome to the land beyond reason.

The son of a mathematician and research engineer, I was raised to believe that problems are for solving. An equal sign in a mathematical equation is the symbol used to communicate, "Here is the answer." With Alzheimer's, there is no right answer. It is a problem without an equal sign or a solution. There is only extending a hand to help, today. And that's where the problem presents itself—will someone answer your call for help? Some people will. Most will not.

For Miss Mary, her closest sister, Peggy, lived on the West coast and had her own health issues. My brother lived in another state. My sister had retired from answering the phone. Marty had her own parent with Alzheimer's. And so it went. When you are the one who is sick, the extended hand is the one you take. It doesn't matter whose it is—even a middle son's or a seven-year-old grandson's hand will do.

2
A Dementia-Friendly Wallet

I remember climbing out of bed one Sunday morning when I was about four, heading downstairs to the living room and finding a different world. A haze of cigarette smoke still hung in the air. Littered on end tables were stinky ash trays, silver bowls of salted peanuts and low-ball glasses holding colorful remains of maraschino cherries, lemon wedges and pimento-stuffed green olives on mini blue swords floating like bathtub toys in stale, murky fluids. I recognized the distinct aroma of whiskey, and it made my head swim as I gobbled up a left-behind mini pecan pie.

The kitchen, normally a hub of activity, sat still and silent. My dad was sleeping past 6:00 a.m. behind a locked bedroom door. He had not made the daily coffee, so the percolator remained asleep, too. Unusual for Mary and Bill, dirty dishes filled the sink, stacked high and precarious. Silver platters, bowls, trays of glasses, long-handled high-ball spoons and squat-handled cheese knives covered the counters. I discovered a stray ham biscuit sitting on a plate, too good to throw away. Waste not; want not.

The furniture in the house had been pushed back to make room for card tables, one after another, perfectly square and covered with green quilted tablecloths that snapped snug around the tabletop's edge. Each table sported an obligatory ashtray and a stack of rectangular aluminum containers about a third of an inch thick that held a perfectly shuffled deck of cards divided into equal parts. My first recollection of Mary and Bill's other lives as contract bridge card sharks.

That morning, considerable cash was piled on the dining room sideboard. Apparently both of them had been on a streak. Miss Mary's girlfriends, Francis and Scotty, later informed me of my mother's bridge skill. "Land sakes! We learned fast that Mary McMullin was not just magazine pretty. She'd cut your balls off before you even knew what happened." Out of survival instinct, you always picked sweet switchblade Mary first.

* * *

Many years later, her girlfriends had a different bridge story to tell me. There were rumors that she couldn't remember cards played. She got confused with the rules of the game. Counting cards was eluding her math mind. Was it her turn? Sweet Miss Mary couldn't remember where she had hidden that switchblade, and she was losing at cards. Behind the magazine-pretty face, her brain was malfunctioning. The protein threads bridging one nerve cell to the next cell were getting tangled and falling down. Like some sick and twisted version of the Mother Goose nursery rhyme, her "neuron bridges were falling down, falling down. Neuron bridges falling down. My fair lady."

Other classic signs of CRS (Can't Remember Shit) emerged. When I opened the door to the attic, there was a stack of unopened Snuggies—the blue blanket with sleeves—ordered from the TV Shopping Network. We already had a lifetime supply of afghan blankets and prayer shawls, compliments of my Great Aunt Vena, a prolific knitter. I didn't think we could use even one Snuggie for the sofa by the TV, let alone a dozen. When I asked who was going to be doing all this snuggling, Miss Mary didn't recall ordering them. We had a SNAFU—Situation SNuggie All Fucked Up.

And when she asked me to pass her a can of tomato soup for lunch, I opened the pantry door and had an Andy Warhol vision. In addition to the Snuggies, we had a dozen cans of Campbell's Tomato Soup perfectly stacked.

"Mom, was tomato soup on super sale?"

"Not that I recall."

"Why do we have so many?"

"Clara and I like it with our grilled cheese sandwich for lunch, Precious."

Miss Mary began to forget recent activities. She was struggling to find words and remember names. She felt confused and forgot to take her daily vitamins and weekly Fosamax. When she went shopping, remembering where she had parked the car became a real issue. But how many times was I myself guilty of wandering through a parking deck hunting for my car and pushing the key-chain remote to locate my honking horn and flashing brake lights?

Despite her mental slip-ups, Miss Mary remained high functioning and adaptable and managed to find a way to get things done for many years. She had lived in her house for so long, she intuitively knew her surroundings. And for decades, the housekeeper came on Wednesdays and kept everything ship-shape. Many families learn their parent has a health problem when the house becomes a mess and falls into disrepair, but Florence kept things scrubbed with permanent scents of Comet Cleanser, Lemon Pledge and Clorox. So symptoms of dementia were masked… for a while. Then something random would occur, like opening the door of the bar to get a lowball glass, and finding the misplaced checkbook and a random can of Campbell's Tomato Soup. Things that make you go *hmmm*… no Bloody Mary was ever made with tomato soup in my father's house.

In her community, Miss Mary was as popular as a rock star. Her fans adored her and were concerned for her well-being. For instance, when I would help my mother with Saturday morning errands and we would enter her neighborhood bank, the tellers and manager would stop what they were doing, turn and greet her from across the room with big smiles, big waves and a big "Hello, Miss Mary!" Brushing me aside, the security guard would personally escort her straight to Katie, her very best friend and bank teller. Her stardom was clear to me—in my lifetime, a teller had never greeted me by name, let alone an entire bank staff. The difference—my mother had time for each fan.

It should have come as no surprise when the bank manager tracked me down and called to share his concern for Miss Mary. He politely reported that she was a favorite customer and seemed to be showing signs of confusion. In fact, she had recently withdrawn a large sum of cash. When he asked about the money, Miss Mary replied with a wink, "Christmas is a time of secrets."

Then her plumber of twenty-five years, Jim, made a special trip to my house to share his concern. Miss Mary seemed disoriented and had tried to pay him twice. He apologized for intruding but said it would break his heart if something happened to her. Jim, her personal plumber and a 270-pound former linebacker, got teary on the subject of Miss Mary's health.

Next, the manager of Ukrop's Super Market—Mike—called me at home. "Mr. McMullin, we are concerned that Miss Mary is carrying quite a lot of cash. She seems to be getting confused at check-out." So many people were looking out for Miss Mary, I felt like I was in the make-believe land of Mayberry with Opey and Aunt Bea.

When my mother had the first health emergency and required the hernia operation, the hospital social worker took one look at me and knew I needed professional help. She connected me to an expert geriatric case worker named Martha Donato to help us with the transition from hospital to home. Martha—the Mary Poppins of senior care—was inordinately fond of Miss Mary and Aunt Clara and described them as "feminists before the word was invented." She agreed to help develop a game plan for our evolving home health care and financial needs. Upon entering our house, Martha Poppins shook my hand and held my elbow firmly. In her experienced and no-nonsense tone, her first comment was, "Keith, falling is the enemy. One fall, and Miss Mary is back in the emergency room with a new set of health problems. The banister on the front stairs needs to be repaired and the pots of geraniums moved off the steps. Today. Please get rid of these throw rugs, especially the one by the stairs. It is a trip hazard, and frankly, if Clara had a bad fall, it could be fatal. You don't have to put the rugs in the garbage can and agitate your mother; just put them out of sight in the attic where she will forget about them."

With an armful of throw rugs, I explained that the banker, plumber and grocery store manager had reached out to me about Miss Mary's confusion with money.

She peered at me above the rim of her glasses. "The good news is that your mother is a special lady. They don't make them like her anymore. The people around her are letting you know—very nicely—that she is manifesting classic signs of Alzheimer's dementia. They are rightfully concerned for her safety. Her banker knows Miss Mary must be protected or she could be taken advantage of as the Millionaire Next Door. Confusion with money is very typical as Alzheimer's progresses from mild to moderate. It is likely that the disease has already advanced through stages one, two and three. Google 'stages of Alzheimer's dementia.' There are helpful websites dedicated to explaining the seven common stages. The time is here for you to talk seriously with her doctor." She then outlined the first phase of a sensible plan of action to begin addressing confusion with money:

1) **One pocketbook** with an easy clasp
2) **One wallet** that is easy to use and easy to take in and out of her pocketbook
3) **One credit card** capped at no more than $1,000 with Power of Attorney paperwork on file at the bank
4) **Front and back copies** of all cards and identification, stored in a file.

So on Saturday after soccer practice, my son and I decided to swing by Grammy Mary's house to implement this prudent care plan. We would go down the list and check things off one-by-one, starting with: **1) One pocketbook with an easy clasp.** I figured the list would take about an hour, and then we would take Grammy Mary to lunch at Bogart's with Legend beer on tap.

James, wearing soccer shorts and cleats, headed upstairs with Grammy Mary to the bedroom. She opened the cedar closet door and began handing him purses. He placed the first one on the bed, then a second, third, a dozen, two dozen, three dozen. The purses covered the queen bed, and I entered a state of shock. I had no idea how to respond to a lifetime of purses.

"This blue one matches spectator pumps."

"I carried the crocodile clutch for years."

The commentary coming out of my mother's mouth was Greek to James and me; we had no idea what spectator pumps were. Thankfully, my son had no problem with this process. One-by-one he turned the purses upside-down and dumped out the artifacts. We made a mountain of lipstick, tissues, change, cards, Certs, bobby pins, ink pens and safety pins. Grammy Mary said magic words. "James, why don't you keep all the money you find for working with me today." Purses flew open.

After a while, Grammy Mary stopped us for lunch, and we ate pimento cheese sandwiches, Mrs. Marshall's potato salad and iced tea. I realized pocketbooks would take all afternoon, and, thankfully, James and Grammy were content to dump and sort. With the Alzheimer's senior, your personal agenda and timeline mean nothing. As James advised, "Slow down the train for Grammy!"

I grew anxious about how we were going to choose one pocketbook from the sea of options. But the assessment was no problem for Miss Mary, "Pass me the black leather one. I wear black flats every day now. Let's not put too much in it; I no longer carry anything heavy." *Perfect.*

The mountain of junk was sorted into hills, including enough lipstick products for all NFL cheerleaders. The stack of cards was three inches thick: credit cards, store cards, library cards, AARP, AAA, A+ Rewards, a grocery store card, one for the gas station, her insurance, etc. Getting her down to one credit card was a task for another day.

We packed the purses into boxes for storage upstairs and out-of-sight. To throw them away right now would create fashion panic. I picked up the funniest one we found, a handbag made of wicker. "Mom, what is this thing? A recycled porch chair?"

She smiled, "Darlin', that's the pocketbook I carried to your wedding, outdoors in summertime. It was a special day. I never dreamed I would have such a dear daughter-in-law."

2) One wallet that is easy to use and easy to take in and out of her pocketbook

When Martha Poppins explained that I needed to take my mother shopping for a dementia-friendly wallet, I knew from personal experience that this was not a good idea for me. I prayed for a modern miracle and dialed my sister who was expert at shopping, but no response. I had thought about asking my wife, but she had her own parent with Alzheimer's to help. I thought about just buying a wallet and giving it to Grammy Mary, but she had absolutely zero faith in my shopping skills and insisted on picking it out herself. So after basketball practice, my son and I drove to Grammy Mary's house, helped her look through the *Richmond Times-Dispatch* for the mandatory Macy's coupons, and loaded in The GramCam—her four-door, four-cylinder, brown Toyota Camry fully un-loaded of any special feature. After I lowered the window with the hand crank, Team Mary took off for Regency Square.

Who knew that Macy's had two separate stores located in the same shopping mall? We finally located Women's Notions & Accessories in Store No. 2, and upon entering, a perky employee sprayed us with cinnamon-scented perfume. Now smelling like Apple Brown Betty, we began searching for a wallet. My mother's case worker had given us the criteria: 1) It must be functional and have easy access to cash, photo ID, credit card, health insurance and Social Security cards. Any other random cards should be removed. 2) A pocket for change was mandatory. 3) All clasps must be easy to open and close. 4) It must fit in-and-out of the pocket-book with ease.

After inspecting a thousand wallets, we began to narrow it down to a handful of hopefuls. My son provided a demonstration of each finalist by putting it in Miss Mary's purse and seeing how easily it came back out. Functionality and ease-of-use narrowed the choices to just two wallets. The black leather one that matched the pocketbook and shoes won. We were ready for checkout!

Upon closer inspection, however, we discovered that the wallet was made by Coach. In the six-point fine print on the coupon, Coach was excluded from the super sale. When we uncovered the price tag hidden inside the box, we found that the wallet cost about the same amount as a fabulous beach vacation. Miss Mary gasped and struggled for air. Coach's overestimated view of its product was a deal-breaker. We would not throw money away on a wallet whose very function was to store money safely. The solution was easy: we were going to Marshall's.

We loaded back into The GramCam and headed across town to Marshall's. As we entered the store, it was apparent that in the world of retail, Marshall's was one step above a yard sale. Miss Mary, our subject-matter-expert on shopping, advised, "Marshall's is a great store if you know what you want, and we do. We are not spending more than $15." My patience was on empty, and what I really needed was a beer. A warm can of Miller Light would be just fine. Luckily, my son was finding the search for a dementia-friendly wallet a generally hilarious misadventure. Like a good Cub Scout, he led Grammy Mary by the hand through the store until we came across women's wallets, all dumped in a bin. I assumed this was how wallets were displayed and sold after falling off the back of a truck on Interstate 95.

Miss Mary and James patiently sifted through the wallets looking for the right combination of function and style. Nothing seemed to suit. James noticed an end-of-the-aisle heap of additional wallets. Saint Anthony, patron saint of all things lost, must have smiled on us, as James pulled the perfect dementia-friendly wallet from the pile. It had all the right compartments and clasps, was just the right size and easy to use. Although it was not exactly the same color as the purse and shoes, it was the same brand and clearly marked $14.98. *Thank you for saving us, Saint Anthony.* We found what had been missing from our lives, and it was on super sale. In humble gratitude, I made a solemn vow never to enter a shopping mall again.

3) One credit card capped at no more than $1,000 with Power of Attorney paperwork on file at the bank

Martha understood working with men and broke things down for me with clear next steps. She prudently advised that when going through my mother's lifetime collection of purses and wallets, I should collect all cards and keep them safe in one place for later.

I had been surprised when my mother, the mathematician, began asking me at check-out, "Now how does this credit card work? Have you already paid it in advance? Who paid the store? When did Visa pay the store? Have we really paid?" The concept of purchasing on credit eluded her sharp mind as dementia gained ground. Martha said that struggling with credit and finances was a classic symptom of Alzheimer's. It was time to limit risk and go with her prescribed plan of one credit card with a maximum credit line of $1,000 and my Power of Attorney paperwork on file with the bank. I trusted Martha Poppins, but little did I realize that she was asking me to take on the credit card industry and capitalism itself.

First, I had to face the three-inch stack of cards. The card on top was tan and written in purple was "LaVogue," not a company I recalled. Miss Mary explained that LaVogue was located downtown and sold fabulous dresses in the 1970s. *I see why we held onto it.* Upon dialing the number, I learned that through countless retail mergers and acquisitions, the account still existed. Dumbfounded, I politely explained that my mother had dementia. She was no longer driving and shopping for cocktail dresses or using credit cards. They explained that, nonetheless, they could not cancel the card, even though it had not been used in thirty years. I explained that I held Power of Attorney and that the medical direction for dementia patients was to limit credit card use. They responded that they could not cancel the card for a medical condition. Corporate policy at its finest.

The only way to cancel my mother's stack of credit cards was for me to take off from work, sit with her at her dining room table during business hours, call each card company and pass the phone to my mother so she could say, "Yes, this is Mary McMullin, and my son is making me cancel all credit cards but one." To which the customer service agent was trained to respond, "Mrs. McMullin, would you like to keep this one?" To which my mother said, "Yes, you have wonderful dresses." And so it went. Her personal mantra: Fashion is always first. The phone came back to me to re-re-explain that my mother has dementia and that we no longer used the card. After a few rounds, Mary conceded and said, "Please cancel my card." One down. One hundred to go.

It was particularly fun when Mary had not used the card in years, and it had a positive balance, a credit to be used. Because we don't waste money, we asked those companies to issue and mail a store gift card. For example, my mother returned something to Lowe's Hardware in 1982 and had a credit of $4.68, enough money for four lightbulbs or four daffodil bulbs. My mother received the store cards, kept them in a rubber band, and we used them prudently for any household purchase, no matter how small the purchase or how far the drive to the store.

Out of the three-inch stack of cards, only our local family-owned bank—First Market Bank—listened attentively and canceled the card politely and efficiently. I loved them for it. Of course since that time, the bank was acquired by a national corporation called Union (not exactly a brand name to inspire consumer loyalty in the South) and has all-new corporate policies based on a pricing spreadsheet likely developed by a twenty-five-year-old with a sparkly new MBA. By nature, Alzheimer's dementia does not fit neatly inside the boxes on any spreadsheet. And as expected, "your mother's health" no longer meets the criteria to cancel Union's bank card.

By dinnertime, we successfully canceled all cards but one. Miss Mary wanted to continue using her CitiBank card. The task was done.

That is, until the following Saturday when I returned to visit. Mary, the dementia patient, had been doing some research into CitiBank. They were increasing the interest rate to 29 percent. Mind you, my mother had never carried a balance on a credit card in her life. She was right, however, they were increasing the interest rate to 29 percent to take advantage of people without the resources to pay off their bill every month. Well-educated crooks. We could do better and find a better credit card company and lower interest rate.

Apparently the answer to our credit card problem was … another credit card. Mary, in her demented state, did some additional research into credit unions. My father once had a Henrico County Federal Credit Union credit card with the interest rate capped at 6 percent. Although he had been dead for several years, she called the credit union, and they were happy to activate the account for her.

So we loaded ourselves into The GramCam and headed to the credit union. We met with the manager, filled out forms, submitted paperwork including Power of Attorney, gained approval, and a new credit card was issued. We were met with a relatively smooth process, that is until we requested the card be capped at no more than $1,000. Miss Mary's measurable value was plummeting. It would take a dozen persistent phone calls, forms and a letter for our request to be approved. Finally, the account was capped at $1,000, and risk was managed for the moment.

4) Front and back copies of all cards and identification, stored in a file

When the new credit card came, I assumed my mother could manage making copies of the VISA, driver's license, health and dental insurance, Medicare and Social Security cards. We needed a copy on file in case we misplaced one of the cards. However, Miss Mary wasn't getting the chore accomplished on her own while I was at work. When I saw her on Saturday morning, she suggested that we do it together. So we drove The GramCam to her neighborhood library to use the copier. Upon entering, the librarian adjusted her glasses with her middle finger, greeted Miss Mary with an excited squeak and emerged from behind the counter for a quick hug. We walked past a plaque with my mother's name engraved on it as a board member of the County of Henrico Public Library when this branch was originally founded. As we stood next to the copier placing cards on the glass face, I watched my mother's large brown eyes and quivering hand. Her expression appeared vacant, and I realized that she couldn't operate a simple machine. And this morning, she did not recall how to use her shiny new credit card either. The times they were a changin' quickly.

3
Problems are for Solving

I remember as a young child, climbing out of bed late at night and heading downstairs to the kitchen. Without saying a word, I would watch my parents through the dining room doorway. Books, yellow legal pads, pencils, an ashtray and Marlboro cigarettes filled the table. My father, the research engineer, and my mother, the mathematician, would sit and solve complex math problems. They both worked the same equation, page after page of calculations spread across the dining room table. In the center of it all sat the pewter Revere punch bowl my father won as golf club champ. Occasionally one of them would look up, take a drag on a cigarette, and say something like, "Pythagorian?" My father would get up from the table, make a Manhattan with Kentucky Gentleman bourbon and sit down to continue the evening of math fun. I've never known anyone else whose parents' relationship involved math intimacy. Thank God they found each other.

In the 1960s and '70s, my mother was a math professor at the University of Richmond. U of R's math department was one of the few open to hiring women at the time. Mom taught courses with names like "Differential Equations" on the men's campus. When possible, she scheduled her classes on Tuesdays and Thursdays to help with the juggle of raising three kids. Florence, our housekeeper, helped with cooking, cleaning, and putting kids down for naps. And she ironed while watching her show, "The Guiding Light." For Miss Mary, every shirt, skirt and pair of Levi's had to be ironed. With starch. No wrinkles. Miss Mary stayed busy as a math teacher and the mother of three kids, and she possessed the desire and the energy to do it all. She was using her gifts.

Her girlfriends stayed at home full time with their kids. Miss Mary thought that sounded like a good idea when my older brother was born one April. However, she missed working and cried every day. Finally in September, the U of R Math Department called and asked if she would consider teaching a couple of calculus courses as they were short-handed and the semester had already started. She hung up the phone, changed clothes, loaded her Bermuda straw bag with textbooks and notebooks, kissed her son, lit a cigarette and drove to campus. They could count on Miss Mary. All in all, she taught math for more than forty years.

Things didn't always go like clockwork. I remember when Florence was sick, and my mother needed to be at the university. Those were the days long before Primrose Day Care or the invention of stay-at-home dads. With three of us running around, she put on a dress, high heels and make-up. It went without saying that a woman in the workforce dressed like a lady, outperformed any man who might want the job and always delivered measurable results. There wasn't wiggle room for error, and she knew it. My mom loved what she did, and any unreasonably high or unfair expectation did not faze her. And if Florence was sick, Mom managed.

This meant that we, too, were dressed in ironed shirts, pants, and jumper, whether we liked it or not. We, too, were loaded into the car, whether we liked it or not. We, too, went to the University of Richmond, whether we liked it or not. With a shoebox full of crayons, we colored and drew and did NOT misbehave in the empty classroom adjacent to Miss Mary's classroom. I could see her through the old wood doorframe. The high ceilings were covered in white asbestos square tiles with small holes about the diameter of a pencil. Florescent light fixtures hung low over wooden desks. Large windows with metal Venetian blinds overlooked the lake. The class was comprised one hundred percent of white men in khakis, loafers and oxford shirts. The majority of her students were majoring in business. Miss Mary stood in front of the enormous blackboard with yellow chalk in hand, the slate covered in mathematical calculations, the room full of raised hands and questions. My mother, in her southern drawl, calmly responded and kept moving forward to solve the next equation. Students took notes and figured math problems with orange number-two pencils in spiral notebooks, young men scribbling to keep up. She ran a fast-moving ship, and some students were left in her wake.

Invariably, one of these students would stray into our classroom. "I see we have a room full of good looking McMullins. If you're half as smart as your mom, you'll be an astronaut for sure. You'll walk on the moon one day." And then he would take us to the blackboard, and we would draw rockets, stars and planets like Saturn with rings. Eventually my mom would come for us. For good behavior, she bought us Cokes in green glass bottles from the faculty lounge refrigerator. Dr. Sherman Grable, head of the math department, would lead us downstairs to the basement to see the model of an electric train encased in glass. And then to the computer room to see an enormous machine covering the walls from floor to ceiling. He would print "punch cards" with our names spelled in small rectangular holes, hanging chads everywhere.

While Dr. Grable showed us the computer, my mom would grade stacks of math tests on legal-sized mimeographed paper, folded long way, with each student's pledge written and signed on the outside: "I have neither given nor received help." Her hand flew as she graded papers with a red Bic pen. She consistently returned the tests the next class period, even if it required that she lose some sleep. Miss Mary was no fool and wasn't about to make it easy for a man to take her job. During my childhood, both of my parents worked. Neither of them ever knew a day of unemployment or underemployment. I recall my father telling me, "If you like your job more days than not, you are fortunate indeed." And indeed, Mary and Bill enjoyed working, enjoyed their careers and each other. As a result, they left their kids a small fortune. The Greatest Generation took care of the next generation, and the next next generation, too.

As long as I can remember, Miss Mary tutored somebody in math. She often met students, including Greg—my football coach from U of R—in Boatwright Library or at our dining room table, and including Aunt Betty, whom my mother helped get admitted into the MBA program. All my life, letters came in the mail to thank her for teaching math and opening the door to a future career. I remember one note on blue paper that read, "Dear Mrs. McMullin, Thank you for patiently teaching Leigh calculus. And thank you for teaching me to believe in my daughter." Sometimes Miss Mary charged a fee, but many times she offered her services for free. She waived the fee if the student's mother was a teacher. She waived the fee if the child was an immigrant and spoke English as a second language. She waived the fee if the parent was divorced or unemployed. She believed in her students. And when I asked why she didn't take money, Miss Mary responded, "I do math. I don't do money."

So much so that she drove over and tutored teenagers who lived at the Virginia Home for Boys, a detention home for juveniles in trouble with the law. Miss Mary taught them all—"black, white, or purple." She didn't care what color the skin, male or female, young or old, rich or poor, criminal record or Boy Scout. I remember being with my father at the country club when one of his golf cronies asked, "Bill, why do you let Mary teach those little felons? It's too risky, far too dangerous." With a laugh, my father responded, "You might be right, but she didn't ask my permission."

Mary skipped grades in school and graduated college with a triple major by about age twenty. She soon found herself teaching kids in Louisville, Kentucky, who were almost her age. Her sister, Peggy, told me of the time when a student opened a switchblade knife to threaten her. Mary, the golf pro, needed only one swing to knock the knife clean out of his hand. She turned his arm behind his back and marched him to the office. The principal wasn't much interested in discipline, but Mary wasn't going to have her class disrupted. If he would do nothing, she would call the police for attempted assault from his desk phone. And that would be the chief of police, her father's old friend and fishing buddy who would respond immediately to Red Compton's oldest daughter. Miss Mary headed back to the classroom and resumed teaching. After that lesson, she didn't face too many more problems with students or administrators. For Miss Mary, problems were for solving quickly.

When I was in high school and college, my buddies referred to my mom as their "math counselor." They would come over for dinner and sit around the table and ask Miss

Mary to heal them of their math wounds. And she would trace back their math injury to the root cause and solve it. A true healer. Some had profound issues with the introduction of a second variable. Others hit a block with factoring. And many simply had never recovered from word problems. Out came the number-two pencil, and problems were addressed once and for all on a cocktail napkin—all before the buzzer rang and blueberry pie emerged bubbling from The Magic Oven. I was bored nearly to the point of death. And after we scarfed down pie, I would try to hustle my buddies out of the kitchen before someone asked the inevitable, "Miss Mary, could you teach me how to play bridge?" And she would respond with a wink, "Sugar, pass the cards. I'll make you an expert." That lesson would last well past midnight.

* * *

Many of us have a Saturday Morning Ritual. As an adult, I like to fantasize that mine involves sleeping late, waking to sex, then a Starbucks Grande Bold and newspaper, followed by bacon and eggs. But the reality is much closer to son's soccer practice, daughter's field hockey game and then yard work, all before lunch. I realized that the sex, coffee and newspaper-in-bed idea is complete fantasy when Miss Mary required a second hernia operation. The procedure was successful, but after being discharged home to recuperate, her geriatric caseworker, Martha, explained that with Miss Mary's declining health and increasing dementia, I needed to help more each week. That's right, I now needed to pay bills and count pills for the brilliant mathematician.

Bills. Review ALL mail, identify and pay bills, save/ organize financial paperwork. Research shows that nearly all seniors with Alzheimer's dementia are taken advantage of financially, often by someone they know—like a greedy relative or neighbor, dishonest home health care nurse or a charity with questionable fundraising practices.

Pills. Fill Miss Mary and Aunt Clara's blue plastic pill-boxes for the home health care nursing aid. Home health care agencies will manage giving medications at the right time, but they do not sort meds and load pillboxes for daily and weekly use. Too many lawsuits (and way too many meds) have restricted the practice.

So our Saturdays began to start earlier, and which-ever child had the first soccer game would go with me to Grammy Mary's to help with the weekly chore of "Bills & Pills." Miss Mary cared exactly nothing about the bills and everything about her grandchild helper. She would answer the door dressed for the day with lipstick applied. She would hug her family, and, in her southern drawl, say, "Precious, I was just thinking about you and making some sweet rolls." And so the Saturday morning ritual began.

Grammy Mary and grandchild would head to the kitchen with gold linoleum flooring circa 1975, open the GE refrigerator, and take out a shiny blue cardboard canister of sweet rolls. Like an ancient Scottish warrior wielding a club, she would raise the tube and wallop the edge of the counter. One loud, startling strike was all it ever took for the rolls to explode from the cardboard. Within seconds, Grammy Mary would have them lined in a century-old baking pan and slid into The Magic Oven. Her grandchild would cheer, "No time for dilly dally!" A rallying cry learned from Miss Mary herself. The required white sugary goop would be stirred and waiting for the moment the hot cinnamon rolls came out of the oven to be "slimed." She would reach into the drawer and get the spoon for sliming and close the drawer effortlessly with her hip, all to the sounds of happy chit and chat. You would think she hadn't spoken with her grandchild since Christmas.

With the cooking demonstration underway, I would tackle additional Saturday chores. First were bills. Martha, advised expertly: "Mary is private about her finances and, unfortunately, can no longer recall financial details. You will need to pay bills for a year to understand exactly what is coming in and what is going out of the house. File in alpha-order every bill and financial paper in a portable, expandable file."

The advice proved expert and essential. For example, who knew my mother had a life insurance policy with Minnesota Life from an employer some forty years ago? Who knew about technology stock my father had bought decades before? Ultimately, we were very fortunate. Miss Mary and Aunt Clara lived well below their means, and, like their thrifty Scottish ancestors of long ago, had saved their pennies for when they would need them. The organized paperwork would prove crucial when my out-of-town brother requested that lawyers review every dime spent.

For the legal financial reporting, the bills essentially fell into five buckets:

1) Household (water, electrical)
2) Credit Card (beauty salon visits, clothing, groceries)
3) Medical (medications, physicians, podiatrist)
4) Financial (bank account, taxes, investments)
5) Gifts (the largest expenses: charity, church, grandchildren presents)

Every Saturday I would go through the bills, write the checks and lay them on the dining room table like a bookkeeper for a CEO. My mom would sit next to me, review the bills and sign. Grandchild-of-the-day would stamp the envelopes, write the return address and add a smiley face sticker for good measure. Accounts payable by committee, done. Most importantly, Team Mary ensured that each bill was paid only once and with the right number of zeros to the left of the decimal. Miss Mary did not really want to be helped, but she really did want to do the right thing. She was a good sport about it and played on the team. One Saturday morning while sitting next to me, she was struggling to balance her checkbook. Despite her concentrated effort, mom could no longer remember how to subtract. She turned and looked at me. "This is the Alzheimer's, isn't it?"

"Yes, it is." And as I sat at the dining room table, I found myself shedding a tear in slow-motion mourning for a U of R math professor I once knew.

Next were pills. Martha Poppins promised me with one hundred percent certainty that my mother was not adhering to her medication schedule. It just wouldn't happen, she said, unless someone else without dementia managed the meds. So each week, I managed a dozen medications for Mary and Clara, sorting them into blue plastic pillboxes labeled with a day of the week and a time of day. First was Aunt Clara's Warfarin to thin and eliminate blood clots. Warfarin came with specific adherence instructions including dosage and diet requirements to effectively keep a person alive. At ninety-eight, Aunt Clara was more concerned with her weekly calcium supplement. "I don't mind being an old lady, but I certainly do not want to be a LITTLE old lady."

Next up were my mother's pills and the sorting of Alzheimer's drugs, which seemed to be all marketing and of no real power. The experts reported that "pharmaceutical science had the worst batting average of all against Alzheimer's dementia. According to the Cleveland Clinic, of the 244 compounds that drug companies tested for the disease over a ten year window, only one received FDA approval. Of the four drugs currently on the market, they were aimed at treating symptoms, rather than curing the disease itself." None-the-less, it was the best we could do in a bad situation. So my mother was prescribed two of the four drugs of questionable value—Aricept and Namenda—and I loaded them into the pill boxes.*

Additional pills were ordered for next time from Westbury Pharmacy. Miss Mary had been shopping at Westbury Pharmacy all my life. The pharmacist greeted her by name, and they delivered her meds to the house at no additional charge. Mary's long-term doctor kept an eye on the multiple prescriptions to ensure that the dosages were correct and there were no negative interactions between medications or unsafe side effects. Medicare and Medicare-supplement insurance paid for the meds. Each week I loaded the pillboxes to ensure they were accurate. Surely we didn't have a medication compliance problem.

But we did have a problem. A big pill problem. The pills did not stay in the bin where they were supposed to be stored in the kitchen. They got moved. Then Mary got confused. Family and nursing aids kept telling Mary to leave the pills alone, but she refused. She was out of compliance. We had worked hard on the daily medication system, but the system was not working. My mother, the straight-A student and sports champion, was failing the team.

One Saturday morning, I noticed the Namenda was missing from the blue plastic bin labeled "Mary." I asked her, "Do you think you might have more Namenda?" I quietly turned and walked behind her. She headed up stairs to the fourth floor, found a key, unlocked the closet, retrieved a crumpled brown paper bag, looked inside and got out another bottle of Namenda. I hazarded a guess, "Is this where you locked pills when we were kids?" "Oh, yes. Your father and I made

* Erika Fry. "Alzheimer's, The Race to a Cure." *Fortune*, May 1, 2015, 80.

sure that pills were out of reach and locked in this closet. You remember Jimmy next door. He nearly died of an accidental overdose and had his stomach pumped. And one time he drank a glass of Clorox. Clean living can kill you!"

Alzheimer's was robbing my mother of short-term memory. She could not recall what the nurse told her yesterday to do with medications. But she walked a familiar path in her mind. She remembered that she put meds in the upstairs hall closet for a good reason. It was both completely rational and irrational. Completely reasonable and unreasonable. Time had evaporated. Alzheimer's was speaking.

Martha made an astute observation to help me understand the mystery of Alzheimer's. She advised us to separate the disease from the person. See the person for who they are, and see the disease for what it is. At first this advice was puzzling, but then it became clear with this issue of medication adherence. Miss Mary was not trying to cause trouble for her family. Rather, Alzheimer's was speaking.

Martha's advice reminded me of a family friend who had died of Alzheimer's. As his dementia progressed, this kind and funny gentleman turned mean, angry and violent. At times he had to be strapped down to his chair to keep from hurting himself or others. The cruel tyrant Alzheimer's had substituted rage for his true personality. In assisted living, he kept leaving his room and walking down the hall and sitting in the last room on the right. Again and again, he left his room and headed down the hall to the same room where he quietly sat in a chair. The staff was at wits end trying to manage his noncompliant behavior and called in a specialist. The psychologist uncovered an answer to the riddle—when he was a boy in New York City, his mother suffered from alcoholism and could be abusive when he came home from school. In their row house, the room down the hall and to the right was the room where he could sit at a desk and study quietly and be left alone. He was seeking a safe and peaceful place. Alzheimer's was speaking.

Miss Mary's primary care doctor, Dr. Gergoudis, had long ago crossed over from the category of medical provider to loyal family friend. He observed that Mary presented the traditional early signs for Alzheimer's dementia, including her family history and a blood biomarker called ApoE. He conducted a series of tests over time that confirmed her mental abilities were declining. But he explained her genius IQ was so high, it could take a long time for her IQ to fall below the normal line and for her to be scientifically classified with mental impairment. From his accumulated volume of experience, she likely had Alzheimer's dementia. However, Dr. Gergoudis explained that an autopsy was the only way to diagnose Alzheimer's with one hundred percent accuracy. (Note: See page 185 for definitions of dementia and delirium.) When we met with the doctor to discuss her dementia, I was the only one upset and teary in the room. Miss Mary had previously self-diagnosed herself with Alzheimer's disease. As Dr. Gergoudis began explaining next steps, Miss Mary smiled and said with a wink, "Thank you, doctor. I'll be sure to drive off that bridge when I get to it."

He observed, "When you have met one Alzheimer's patient, you have met exactly one Alzheimer's patient." The human brain is so complex and intricate, that as Alzheimer's disease begins to deteriorate brain cells and nerve endings, an infinite number of variations of mental loss and dementia can present in the patient. The middle layer of the brain, the hippocampus, is typically the first area to be impacted. This is the area of the brain linked to memory, personality, and emotion, exactly what makes each of us uniquely human. The disease was attacking the part of my mother's brain that made her uniquely Miss Mary. And she had begun to struggle with senses... and not just her sense of fashion. Her sense of smell had declined, and taste was right behind it. She had begun asking her grandkids to sniff and taste-test the stuffing and to advise her if it needed more sage or pepper. Her eyesight was getting worse, and she had begun to complain of double vision while watching TV. Hearing remained intact, but she was having spells of vertigo, linked to the inner ear. Miss Mary was taking leave of her senses.

4
Drive You Crazy

I remember when cars were large and consumed huge volumes of cheap gasoline to keep their V8 engines churning. They were a celebration of automotive obesity. Land-yachts. Sedans. Roadmasters. Gas guzzlers. Ours was a Ford Fury. Very big, very brown, four doors and seated about twenty comfortably. My father once loaded a table and two chairs into the trunk, closing it easily. The advantage of a Ford Fury for a family of five was that three kids could sit in the backseat, and no one actually had to touch each other. On a road trip, every person had ample space to lounge and sleep and stare out the window. If you ever did cross the line and actually touch someone, a sharp jab moved you back across the boundary line marked by stitches in the vinyl upholstery and into your defined territory. "Jab-Jab-Punch" was how it went.

I remember sitting on the black vinyl bench seat, zoning, a hundred percent bored, head resting against Old Bunny— still reliable despite some stuffing and mesh coming out the ears—watching and counting cows and horses, farms and power lines as they went by on Interstate 64. Every summer in July, we drove hundreds of miles west from Richmond, Virginia, to Lexington, Kentucky, on Family Vacation. The road trip took about fourteen hours, each way. And this was well before Steve Jobs invented the Apple in his garage—so we had no iPod, no iPhone, no iPad, no DVD players, no digital anything. Just miles and miles of black asphalt road with its white dotted line unfolding before us in the stifling heat of July.

My good-looking mom sat in the passenger seat. She looked right out of a Pall Mall cigarette ad, with her Bermuda shorts, black sunglasses, crossed tan legs and bare feet. I watched as she reached for another cigarette and placed it between her lips. She would push the round lighter into the dash, and when it popped white hot, she lit, took a drag and exhaled with an easy confidence. I knew exactly how that lighter worked having tested it once. I put my finger in it to touch the coil and burned off the tip of my finger. White hot. Burnt flesh smell. Never did that again.

Land-yachts came with many features, including a small triangular window on the door of the front seats. Opened slightly and similar to a sail, it caught the wind and served as an air vent. The perfect accessory for a smoker, my mom expertly used this window-vent to ash her cigarette and exhale smoke to the outside world. She gazed forward as another hundred miles passed.

My parents began each day of driving by singing a rousing version of their jazz standard "We're on our way; We're on our way!" Time on the road was measured by meals. My dad would wake us before the sun rose and carry my sister to the car. Too tired to fight, we fell back asleep while he drove for several hours before stopping for breakfast at a diner or IHOP. International House of Pancakes. Who knew that pancakes were a diabetes taste treat around the globe? All we wanted was out of the car, to stand up, to stretch. My father would quickly order a cup of coffee. Mary would light a cigarette—the perfect side to the day's first cup of coffee.

Once loaded back in the Ford Fury, my father would have his right hand on the steering wheel and his left arm resting on the door panel. He was as steady as they came and, without complaint, would drive all day until we reached his mother's house in Lexington. A member of "The Greatest Generation," Bill worked as an engineer in Research and Development for Reynolds Metals Corporation. Like the aluminum products he designed, Bill was durable, dependable and high functioning. My father was exactly who you wanted on your team, and he worked at Reynolds for more than thirty years until he retired with a generous pension, which my parents saved in its entirety. The Greatest Generation was also The Long Lost Generation. He worked hard each day and did right by The Company. In turn, The Company did right by him and helped take care of his family in retirement.

Of course when we traveled, my Dad was on "paid vacation." And with him at the wheel, there was nothing to worry about, unless you caused trouble. If you generated a back seat problem, the right hand of justice flew at lightning speed over the top of his seat and delivered a whack to straighten things out and get you back in line. No backseat quarreling ever escalated out-of-control on his watch.

As we drove through the mountains of West Virginia, the highways turned into byways that wound through the Appalachian Mountains. Most trips, one child would start feeling queasy and be moved to the front seat between my parents and be given clear instruction to look straight ahead out the windshield at the horizon line. Eventually, Bill would pull off the road for a break at a mountain swimming hole, an ancient waterfall rumbling over coal black rocks and dumping spring water into a pool. It was far too cold to wade in. You had to hurl your body in, taking a polar bear plunge. Too frigid to scream, all you heard was the sound of a swimmer surfacing and the gasp for air from a wide-open mouth. Fingers, toes, lungs, penis—everything blue. No one could ever stay in the mountain pool longer than a few minutes. I would climb out shivering with goose bumps, dry off in a towel, put on dry clothes and jump back in the car. The black vinyl seats warmed shivering legs.

My father could drive the mountain roads of West Virginia with just one hand on the wheel and little braking. He wasn't the type to flinch. West Virginia storms were legendary for rolling over the ridge and surprising drivers with a mountain monsoon. It could be blue sky one minute, and then in a flash, so dark you could barely see the hood of the car. Our windshield wipers would be maxed out, the rain sounding like pebbles hitting the roof. The roads would be lined with cars pulled over, red hazard lights flashing S.O.S. My father, however, would move to the left lane and keep moving forward. "Just a little rain," he deadpanned, single hand on the wheel guiding us around curves, over hills. We drove through the edge of the storm as if exiting a car wash, instantly emerging onto dry land with no sign of rainwater or need for wipers at hyper speed.

Eventually, we would cross the state line into Kentucky and be back on Interstate 64 heading to Lexington. Full speed ahead, he drove that Ford Fury well above the seventy-five miles per hour speed limit. On the outskirts of Lexington, my father would announce, "We are there yet." With shouts of liberation from the backseat, my mother would open her purse and expertly apply red lipstick and comb her dark hair. Fourteen hours in the car with three kids in 90-degree heat could not damage her easy good looks. At long last, we would turn left onto Millbrook Drive and pull up to my grandmother's familiar red brick house with the Mimosa tree in the side yard covered in pink fuzzy blooms like something out of Dr. Seuss. Mom Mom, wearing an apron and sitting on the front porch, would be waiting for us while she passed the time by shucking Silver Queen corn and snapping green beans into a white enamel basin. Mistah Kitty was by her side purring and wrapping his grey tail around her slim leg. It felt like we had been gone about ten minutes to run an errand to the store, rather than an entire school year.

For my dad, visiting Mom Mom included "Billy's List." All year she kept a list on a lined pad of all things needing to be fixed. With me as mechanic's assistant to pass him the Philips head screwdriver, one-eighth inch drill bit, ratchet or hack saw, he went about Mom Mom's house repairing all things broken: screen doors, toaster oven, bathroom sink, dresser drawer, basement drain. The reward for being Mr. Fixit: a feast for dinner. And it was good training for me. Little did I know that one day managing lengthy to-do-lists for my mom would be an invaluable skill as her dementia progressed.

Of all the relatives to visit, none was more fun than Uncle Bob. Outside of Lexington, we would pull off the main road, open the gate to his horse farm and drive up the twisting gravel driveway to the brick colonial house on top of the hill. A big man with an impressive belly, Uncle Bob always greeted us in jeans and cowboy boots with a big "How-do!" Uncle Bob's idea of farming was more like Noah than Ole McDonald. Indulgent, he owned two of almost everything: two chickens with hair, two chickens that laid green eggs, two red hens that laid blue eggs, two llamas, two sheep, two ostriches, two sons, two dozen cats and dogs, too many horses, but only one goat named Zeke. No need for more goats—this one consumed all things, including the shirt off my back. One afternoon, I stood there dumbfounded and bare-chested as he devoured the shirt right off me. I learned fast to keep a safe distance from the beast called Zeke.

My cousin Betsy knew the farm like the back of her hand and how to have fun with suburban cousins. In no time, she would lead us to the horse barn. Betsy said it would be a good idea for me to ride a stallion named Ringo Star.

"What about Paula the pony?"

"Nah, Ringo is just right for you."

I saddled up and followed Betsy out of the barn, across the farm, through woods and by ponds with enormous bullfrogs. Bored playing tour guide, she turned Ringo just enough for his eye to catch sight of the barn. Ringo lurched wildly and ran in full gallop toward it with me holding on tight to the saddle horn, laughing my head off. As we raced uphill, my ass bumping all over the saddle, I heard Uncle Bob shout from the porch a stern one-word command, "Duck!" And in the nick of time, I ducked my head and just missed getting it knocked clean off my shoulders by the beam above the barn door. For my cousins, this beat the hell out of listening to bullfrogs.

Uncle Bob was a man of great excess, full of life. The barn. The animals. The garden with exotic imported plants. He ran a fantasy farm, complete with swimming pool, ping pong, pool table, air hockey and foosball. Even his office where I slept was entertaining, his stash of *Playboy* mags in the bottom cabinet.

Amidst these fond memories is another image etched just as vividly in my mind. I remember passing the blue living room. Stopping. Looking through the doorway. It was not really a living room but rather a dying room. Full of medical equipment and a hospital bed in the center, my grandmother's slim body lay twisted beneath a white sheet, like a mature butterfly that had been crumpled back inside its white cocoon. A metal crane-like apparatus positioned over the bed assisted in moving her body. It was impossible to believe she weighed more than a hundred pounds. Uncle Bob described her as a "vegetable," conjuring up images in my mind of eggplant, squash or rhubarb with my grandmother's face, her nose a stem. They said Grandmother Jewel had Alzheimer's disease. She lay in the bed all day, staring and not speaking, no longer able to engage with her four daughters surrounding her, each as strikingly beautiful as the next. My mother would sit next to her for hours, her hand resting on her mother's arm. That blue room was the only quiet place on Uncle Bob's horse farm where the air was still.

My family has always lived in the shadow of Alzheimer's dementia. For more than 100 years it has been reducing loved-ones to vegetables in the garden of good and evil. Some research scientists publish theories that Alzheimer's is really "Diabetes Type 3" or "diabetes of the brain" that potentially could be treated with lifestyle changes like a Mediterranean low-carb diet and medication. While interesting, for people like me who have experienced generations of healthy relatives slowly wasted by the disease, it seems highly improbable that there is no genetic link or hereditary risk factor.

Between my family and my wife's, the list is long of people who have suffered with Alzheimer's: Grandmother Jewel, Great Grandfather Caloway, Great Aunt Kate, Aunt Sarah, Uncle Charlie, Bampaw, Bammaw, Louise, Jo Jo. In a particularly cruel twist of fate, my mother, Miss Mary, and my father-in-law, Ole Daddy, were both dying of it at the same time, both requiring more and more care as their minds deteriorated. It is likely that my wife and/or I will die of Alzheimer's. Deciding to buy long-term care insurance for each of us was easy as rhubarb pie. My prayer is that it will be Aunt Kate's type, where you exist delusional and happy, completely unaware that you are blowing through half a million dollars on health care that can't cure you.

On Uncle Bob's farm, Mother Nature taught me many things about life. Surrounded by animals, birds, plants and insects, I learned the cycle of sex, birth, life and the struggle to survive. I watched baby chickens hatch from the egg in the morning and Mr. Hawk swoop down and snatch them for a midday snack. Later in the day, I gobbled down Aunt Elizabeth's seriously good fried chicken—Mama Chicken— and deviled eggs made from her unborn babies. On Ringo Star, I learned the challenges of my own survival and narrowly escaped a violent beheading. And I observed life in the retention pond. I saw frogs devour water bugs skating across the pond's surface. I watched baby-brother tadpole graze on slimy pond grass and become a snack for Mr. Cat Fish emerging from the muck. By the light of the moon, I watched in disbelief as cousin Bud followed the croaking sound of a bull frog and purposefully shined his flashlight directly in its eyes. Temporarily blinded, he then gigged Kermit with a pitchfork, apparently on loan from the devil. With his knife, he sliced off the still-twitching green frog legs to fry until crispy in a skillet swiped from his mother's kitchen cabinet. No one was safe. I was experiencing Mother Nature firsthand, a mother who didn't play fairly or give second chances. She could be a stone-hearted bitch and devour her young. Mother Mary was the one who taught me the nature of love, forgiveness and to extend a hand to your own dying mother.

* * *

Every summer of Mary and Bill's married life together, they drove home to Lexington to visit their families. About ten years before I was born, my father—the engineer—wrote a story following their trip and mailed it to *The Reader's Digest* for consideration to be published. Below is his submission to the editor of the section called *Life in These United States:*

Dear Editor:

NEVER UNDERESTIMATE THE POWER OF MARY

During summer vacation, my wife Mary and I visited our hometown of Lexington, KY—a mid-size town of about 100,000 people. During our trip, we were having some trouble starting our car. For some unknown reason, when trying to start it a solenoid switch in the ignition system would stick and the car motor would not turn over. But it is really a simple matter to start the car… if you know how. Thinking that sometime Mary might have trouble when alone, I showed her how to start it just in case.

Once back at home, my wife decided to drive downtown to do some shopping. Wearing a dress and hat, she got her purse and white gloves and drove downtown. She parked in a valet parking garage. Upon returning some time later from shopping, the attendants told her that they could not start the car and had to push the car to its parking spot. At first they thought it was the battery, but the horn worked and the lights burned brightly. They thought it was out of gas and put gas in the car, but it still would not start. Mary apologized for the inconvenience, paid and thanked them. She held out her hand for the keys, ignoring their sideways glances.

She walked back to the car with the three attendants following to help. The men's snickering turned into laughing as she took off her white gloves and raised the hood. They laughed louder when she reached down and picked up a rock. As they watched, Mary took the rock and firmly tapped the solenoid, then got in the car and started it on the first try. She lowered the hood, put on her gloves, and drove off as their look of amusement turned into utter astonishment at the power of Mary.

As fate would have it, the power of Mary began to fade as she started showing more signs of Alzheimer's disease. With her increasing dementia, I did not want to overestimate her driving ability. For years, Grammy Mary had been driving The GramCam. She liked nothing more than to load up her grandkids—Charlotte, James, Emily and Caroline—and head to the Science Museum or IMAX Theater with her dutifully saved white envelope of member passes for free admission. From the backseat of The GramCam, Charlotte would command, "Next stop: Santa Barbara!" Grammy Mary laughed. "Aye-aye, Captain. Buckle up." Other than edu-tainment for the grandkids, Miss Mary's driving primarily took her to Ukrop's Super Market, Westbury Pharmacy and Mary Lou's Hair Salon, all within a couple miles of her house.

But when she drove herself to the emergency room, Dr. Scream made it clear that things needed to change. Even with limited driving and a flawless driving record, a senior behind the wheel with dementia and vertigo was cause for alarm. Mom's lawyer suggested I Google the names of her Alzheimer's drugs and read about multi-million dollar lawsuits against seniors taking these medications who had been involved in car accidents. Our trusted advisor, Dr. Gergoudis, politely explained that his own father had stopped driving, and he was in better health than Miss Mary. His father had stopped driving because he didn't want to risk causing injury to someone else.

Dr. Gergoudis recommended Miss Mary take a driving test from a medical professional called an occupational therapist (OT). In his experience, my mom's generation listened to a doctor-type far more readily than to their own children. After all, a parent tells a child what to do and not the other way around. This was especially true for matriarchal figures like Miss Mary. If they failed the test, the medical professional would suspend the driver's license with DMV and the emotional battle with a child would be avoided. Dr. Gergoudis observed that losing permission to drive is often the change with the single-greatest impact on an aging senior because the loss of the driver's license is proof of growing older, dependency and losing control. It can feel like a punishment of isolated confinement. He suggested I take an additional family member with me to avoid getting lambasted personally. I asked, but my siblings were far too smart to get involved. Instead of helping, they wanted a follow-up report by email, including an estimated value of the Camry. I was reminded that The GramCam did not belong to me but to my mother and her estate. You would have thought that I was being paid to assist my mom. I was growing road weary of the daydream that Miss Mary's children would play together nicely. Like in the backseat of the Ford Fury, we each stayed in our defined territory marked by stitches in the vinyl upholstery, and if you crossed the line and touched, Jab-Jab-Punch.

Miss Mary, the straight-A student, got a copy of the DMV driver's education book and began studying. Despite

Alzheimer's dementia, she was determined to pass. The night before, she stayed up until 2:00 a.m. reviewing questions and answers. The next day, she got dressed and looked her best as we headed to the medical center for the test. An old pro, the occupational therapist administered the test while I waited on a deacon's bench in the hall. In less than thirty minutes, she brought Miss Mary to sit beside me, and with practiced skill, said, "Miss Mary, you are a remarkable woman. I hope to be like you—so engaged and poised. You got the right answer to each question. However, your response time was too slow. With driving, response time to react to other drivers is very important. And although you were able to answer the questions correctly, it took more time than the test allows. You did not pass."

The two spoke some more. Miss Mary was in shock and listened more than she talked. It was the first test she had ever failed in life, even if she failed by the clock and not by the subject matter. I choked up, and tears flowed down my cheek. As we stood to leave, Miss Mary turned to me and said all that remained to be said, "I sure could use a drink. Make mine a double, Pussycat." We drove back to my house, and we had a drink on the patio. Mom and my wife chatted about everyday things—kids at camp, the virtues of red geraniums versus coral or pink, sandals on sale in the Lucky Lady Room at Saxon Shoes, spinach lasagna for dinner. Like after a funeral and great personal loss, Miss Mary instinctively moved on to the next thing and began adjusting to a new normal.

During the weekend, I was required to put a lockbox in her house with the car key inside for only the nurse or driver to access. I anticipated my mom being upset and difficult. But Miss Mary was composed. She had already said goodbye to driving The GramCam and had adjusted to a new normal. "You know my mother didn't drive, except when Aunt Linda played the oboe in the All-City Orchestra."

"Aunt Linda played the oboe?"

"Yes, she's the only one of us who got any of Grandmother's musical ability."

"Your mother drove her to music practice?"

"And to performances across town. Mother's fear was learning to drive. My fear was stopping to drive. She taught me to face my fears."

And my fear was an accident and lawsuit for millions of dollars. We all kept moving forward on this unmarked road.

5

The Kayak Method

"Too much to do" is the uncontested leader of the pack of sources for caregiver stress. The additional most common stressors identified by the doctors at the Mayo Clinic are:

2) Added responsibilities
3) Frustrations of daily care
4) Changes that impact your lifestyle
5) Feeling inadequate
6) Personal loss or grief
7) Disagreements regarding care
8) Uncertainty about the future[*]

I maxed out this entire list of stressful feelings just trying to help Miss Mary find a dementia-friendly wallet. That

---

[*] Ronald Petersen, M.D., Ph.D., ed. *Mayo Clinic Guide to Alzheimer's Disease: The Essential Resource for Treatment, Coping and Caregiving.* Rochester, MN: Mayo Clinic Health Information, 2006, 250–253.

experience alone was completely overwhelming and moved me entirely out of my happy place. And nowhere in the Mayo Clinic Health Information's special purple section labeled *Action Guide* did it mention what to do when your mother's Aunt Clara is added to the caregiving mix. And feelings of suicide, homicide and euthanasia are definitely omitted from the resource guide.

But there is a section headed *Learn to Relax*. As I was getting busier and busier with caregiving, that sounded very good. The doctors suggest you "develop a strategy that can help you relax whenever you find yourself becoming stressed."* Continuing to read, the key recommendation is for diaphragmatic breathing (a.k.a. deep breaths). Other suggested techniques are muscle relaxation, visualization, autogenic relaxation, hypnosis and meditation. With Jerry Seinfeld as my spiritual guide on TV, I tried closing my eyes like Frank Costanza and repeating "Serenity Now!" whenever I felt my blood pressure climbing. My adopted mantra of "Serenity Now! Serenity Now!" at least brought on a good laugh. Then I realized that I actually do know something about serenity, breathing and meditation—I just call it kayaking.

* * *

When "too much to do" is the daily guarantee, kayaking begins before dawn and before Abner the barking beagle sounds his wake-up call. Lying in bed, I could hear my father's voice inside my head with the sailor's order of the day: *Feet on the floor!* Rolling back the covers, my bare legs and feet left the warmth of the bed and touched cold oak

---

* Ronald Petersen, M.D., Ph.D., ed. *Mayo Clinic Guide to Alzheimer's Disease: The Essential Resource for Treatment, Coping and Caregiving.* Rochester, MN: Mayo Clinic Health Information, 2006, 251.

floorboards. Careful not to make any noise that would wake Marty, my hand found the all-important eye glasses on the nightstand. Waking my wife this early would only result in creating additional stress… divorce had happened over far less. Walking quietly across the dark room with my left knee complaining about each step, I found my swim trunks. Boxers dropped, me shivering cold, I pulled them on, the mesh liner uncomfortably tight. Quickly putting on an old gym t-shirt and fleece, my feet would find their familiar river sandals, the straps encrusted in river mud.

I walked quietly down the stairs and made a cup of instant coffee. Good enough before the friendly morning shift started at Starbucks on River Road. While the Highlander warmed up, I shot a text to early-riser Doug to see if he wanted to kayak or fish. But duty called with the kids. "nxt time. thx." I drove across the Huguenot Bridge, the James River barely visible in darkness. I unlocked the camouflaged gate at Jones Landing, rolled it open wide enough for the SUV to drive through and park. I lifted the neon green Jackson kayak from the boat rack and rolled it onto my back, turtle like, the cold shell against my shoulders and neck.

In the early morning light, the fresh water of the James moved at a fast clip over the rocks I needed to avoid. Fastening my life preserver, I lowered the kayak from the dock to the water's surface and slid in, freezing my ass off in the hard plastic seat. With paddle in both hands, I took a stroke and moved to the middle of the river. I would not be cold for long.

I paddled upstream against the current as morning light painted a watercolor sky. I paddled through rising morning steam. Stately great blue herons patiently fished and watched me paddle by. With no signs of another human being, I was the sole owner of this James River waterfront. King David and Great Aunt Clara whispered their song:

The heavens declare the glory of God;
the skies proclaim his handiwork.

Day after day they pour forth speech;
night after night they reveal knowledge...

								Psalm 19

At the bend before the Willey Bridge, the water smoothed. I sat perfectly still in the kayak and took ten slow strokes in rhythm with ten deep breaths, focusing on the paddle entering the water and the ripples it sent out. As I paddled toward Bosher's Dam, the river's current strengthened, as did each stroke I made, using only my arms and holding my body and kayak still to maximize efficiency and speed. As the James River poured over the dam in a powerful waterfall, I hung back about four feet from the waterfall's edge to prevent being sucked down into the mighty vortex. A bald eagle fished the dam without fear, singing his male soprano song. He flew directly at the river, and, with precision, snatched a small mouth bass in his right yellow talon. Large black wings unfurled and with a flash of white tail-feathers, he raised above the water and perched on the branch of a dead tree to eat this morning's catch; his watchful yellow eye making sure I kept my distance.

I paddled back downstream to the dock, back to the daily business of living, back to the balancing act of career, spouse, kids and my mother struggling with Alzheimer's dementia. There was nothing easy about shoehorning "senior caregiving" for Miss Mary and Great Aunt Clara into daily life. The approach I took to caregiving focused on doing one thing each day for them—a phone call to the doctor, an insurance check deposited, a prescription ordered. It was what I knew how to do from rowing. Every day I put the paddle in the water and took one stroke. Kayaking required steady strokes, one after another, and each stroke has a slight course correction to keep the boat headed in the right direction. I knew with a competitive job in health care and technology, kids, and a wife with her own parent with Alzheimer's, The Kayak Method was what I could manage, and this approach brought a piece of peace amidst the turbulent swirling water on this unchartered river. The "Drop Everything to Help!" emergency approach wasn't realistic for me. I would lose my job, putting my own family in crisis and humiliating Mary and Clara. But I could set an ongoing rhythm, like paddling to shore. I could reach out my hand and do one thing to help her every day.

I had awoken from the team dream and stopped expecting help or asking for a hand from my brother and sister. Martha Poppins assessed that there are really three types of people. 1) Some people don't say they are going to do anything, and they don't. 2) Some people say they are going to do things, and then don't do them. 3) Some people just do things. Martha observed that my distant brother would not be helping, and my sister would help sometimes, as long as it was to her liking. She felt the single most valuable contribution that Libby could make would be attending doctor appointments with mom to hear what the doctor had to say. Four ears are better than two, and especially in the case of a dementia patient. It would not be easy to coordinate, but Martha volunteered to try reaching her.

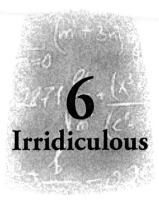

6
Irridiculous

Monday morning I was back at the office and packing my laptop to travel to the Indianapolis HQ for a full day of meetings on Tuesday. It looked like half a day of connecting flights to get there. The purpose of the meeting was to integrate disease prevention and management into the overall strategic plans of Blue Cross and Blue Shield across the country. A noble health care goal.

As I talked with the team of marketing and program managers before leaving for the airport, my cell phone vibrated. A nurse at Henrico Doctor's Hospital was calling because Clara Napier had been taken by ambulance to the emergency room and admitted for acute pain. She was not stable and was being transferred to the Intensive Care Unit (ICU). I looked at my watch and calculated that if I left then, I could swing by the hospital, talk with the doctor and Miss Mary, jump on the interstate and drive directly to the airport. I could attend the meeting in Indy and be back home late Tuesday night. My prayer: *God of the Universe, please let there be a parking spot in the front lot by the door.*

As I signed in at the ICU and headed to room 231, the nurse stopped me outside the door. Aunt Clara had delirium and was hallucinating. She was not staying in her hospital bed. She was not keeping the IV in her arm. And Miss Mary was not at the hospital, but rather, she was lying down at home with vertigo. She was having another spell. The nurse asked who had the medical directive for Aunt Clara to make the medical decisions necessary for the doctor to provide for her care. My mother was no longer qualified.

In my best Doctor-on-TV voice, I said, "Medical Directive. What do you need, exactly?"

The nurse explained that I needed the legal document for Aunt Clara that identified who could make health care decisions for her. The delirium she was experiencing might have been brought on by stress or fever, which meant she might come out of it. But she might not. She was very sick and had blood clotting in her lungs. If one blood clot traveled to her heart, her life could end in seconds. Her medical directive, the nurse explained, should be with her other legal papers.

I did not bother driving home to rummage through files. The reason my great aunt had lived to age ninety-eight was because she had been healthy and strong all her life. She had probably been in a hospital once or twice before. I vaguely remembered when she tripped on a stair and broke her arm about thirty-five years before. And if she did have a medical directive, there was no way it would name me, one of a cast of a thousand nieces and nephews.

The nurse explained that we could call our lawyer to come to the hospital and draw up a new medical directive in the hospital room. Hopefully there would be a time when she was lucid and could sign it. With Miss Mary experiencing dementia-related vertigo, the nurse explained that she would not qualify. At that moment, I was positive that I was the one with vertigo and was stuck in some sort of spin-cycle from hell. It was looking like it would be an afternoon of doctors AND lawyers, a formula for the most expensive afternoon of my great aunt's ninety-eight years.

I was pacing the hall and anxious with the realization that I was not getting on a plane and going anywhere to *talk about* health care. I would be *practicing* health care right where I was standing instead. Fortunately like my aunt, I rarely got sick and had months of accumulated sick leave. However, I was a team member you could count on. I wasn't in the habit of skipping meetings, bailing on presentations, giving excuses or dropping the ball. I feared exposure and that coworkers would discover my invisible double-life as a senior caregiver. If people at the office had any idea of the volume of caregiving that I shouldered, they could rightfully question my commitment to the day job. And they could rightfully question my sanity. Uneasy, I called my manager's cell phone to explain the family health emergency. The boss responded, "Anything to get out of that flight to Indy!" I laughed at the joke and breathed a heavy sigh of relief. This corporate boss got the rare A+ in compassion.

I hung up and headed into Aunt Clara's room. She recognized me immediately... and recognized all sorts of imaginary people in the room with us, too. I sat with her, my hand on her arm. Her hallucinations were happy with children coming and going. She was delirious and living in a dream world of her own making. She was always smart, and a dream world far surpassed the cold reality of the ICU.

I knew two things for certain. First, taking care of Aunt Clara with delirium at the hospital and Grammy Mary with dementia at home required more than just me. Second, if corporate America had taught me anything, it was how to recruit and motivate a team of professionals to be successful. Amidst the crazy chaos, I instinctively started building the team:

1) Clara's nurse said that we needed a **case worker**, and Martha Poppins magically appeared at Clara's door. Was I hallucinating, too? I halfway expected her to be carrying a carpet bag and umbrella. She became the single-most important person in our chaotic world. I thought of Martha as a quarterback of care, anchoring our team. She wielded her cell phone like a corporate CEO and skillfully connected us to the right players— experts on legal needs, hospital discharge, rehabilitation and Medicare. Most importantly, she genuinely cared for Clara and focused on her as a person. There was no hiding true compassion.

2) We needed **home health care.** Dawn Benninghove with Companion Extraordinaire Home Health Care had previously evaluated my mom and Aunt Clara and now came to our rescue. In a flash, Dawn lined up a nurse to stay overnight with my aunt in the ICU as required by the hospital to prevent injury or accident while she was hallucinating and wandering. Dawn lined up another professional to help my mom at home in bed as she was too sick to stand. She began developing a schedule for when my aunt was discharged to help her and Mary. With Dawn and Martha, I began filling out paperwork for Medicare and insurance to help pay for all of this required care.

3) Martha introduced me by phone to Paul Izzo, a top **estate attorney**. He guided me through the maze of medical directives, power of attorney, wills and estate settlement. Like Martha, Paul focused first on my aunt and her needs.

4-6) **Doctor, Lawyer, Indian Chief.** We now had the doctor, care team and lawyer that we needed. We had most everything for the moment, except for that elusive Indian Chief. Fortunately, after a good night's sleep, Great Aunt Clara rallied. Her delirium was short lived, and she returned to the here and now. I knew we were in a far better place when she requested that her hair be washed and set. With her good looks restored, she thanked the doctors and nurses for their time and expert opinions about her pulmonary embolism. She agreed to take their recommended generic prescription that was covered by her Medicare policy. She then declined all additional testing and further medical procedures as unnecessary. She began helping with the logistics for her discharge to go home. With the medical team, Clara politely and clearly shared, "I'm not afraid to die." The Indian Chief had spoken.

* * *

Once Clara transitioned home and her health began to improve, I found myself promoted to power of attorney for both Mary Compton McMullin and Clara Ethel Napier. Make mine a double, pussycat, to celebrate this battlefield promotion. I needed to add financial expertise to the team to help with the business side of senior caregiving:

7) expert **financial advisor** experienced with estates
8) smart **tax accountant**
9) detail-oriented **paralegal** within Paul's law firm to help with financial reporting.
10) a sassy **real estate agent** would be needed in time. However, the reality was that my siblings would not like anyone I chose. Aunt Clara observed that it wasn't

possible for me to make them happy. So we muddled through an insane power game of two-kids-against-one. My brother and sister frustrated my mother's caseworker so much with emails about finances written in a threatening tone that eventually she fired us as her client. Martha Poppins wasn't one to be trifled with, and one day she would disappear from our lives as quickly as she had appeared. She loved and respected Miss Mary but advised that we likely required a lawyer to manage our family.

Martha's recommendation in rank order was: 1) family counseling, 2) mediation, 3) lawyer. Exactly as anticipated, my siblings immediately declined options one and two, and "working together" was swept off the table. So we called in Miss Mary's lawyer, Paul Izzo. Undoubtedly, we were not the first—nor the last—family to be managed by a lawyer. Like looking through the lens of a microscope at cells impacted by Alzheimer's dementia, our weaknesses were being magnified. Each of us was malfunctioning, and our connection to one another was breaking down. It embarrassed Miss Mary that her family needed a lawyer, and she described the situation as "irridiculous"—a hybrid of "irrational" and "ridiculous." A brilliant dementia slip-up. My brother, sister and I were now managed by the law firm of ThompsonMcMullan and permanently branded "the troubled children."

In addition to the core team it took to manage a senior with Alzheimer's, there were some friends and family members who offered help. My theory was to open the door wide and let them assist in whatever way they wanted, as long as there was no safety concern. If someone wanted to take Miss Mary to get her hair done or to church or to have lunch at the Club, I welcomed it. A sad reality for me and my wife was that her father, Ole Daddy, was dying of Alzheimer's dementia at the same time as Miss Mary. And simultaneously, we each had an aunt dying of Alzheimer's. This disease is a hyper-absorber of resources—energy, time, money, emotion, life itself.

My wife's parents lived happily-ever-after in separate houses located next door to each other. Although they lived side-by-side, Martha assumed the responsibility of taking care of my sick father-in-law, Ole Daddy, when his Alzheimer's disease began to progress. She did not turn to her children to manage his care but took on the responsibility herself. She found the doctors, located the assisted living facilities, and made the daily decisions for health care. I felt my wife's role was to help her mom as much as she would allow. My father-in-law enjoyed an out-of-town girlfriend for years, but no surprise, she vanished when Alzheimer's appeared. To some, it was pretty outrageous that his neighbor wife would cook him dinner, let alone manage his care for Alzheimer's dementia, but she kept her marriage vow to the letter of the law—in sickness and in health. While she managed his care, her oldest son (a.k.a. Uncle Gus) managed the finances, the two big buckets of what it takes to provide care for a senior. My mother and father-in-laws' relationship may have been non-traditional, but it functioned far better than most when it came to caregiving for dementia. Martha's words of caution—"If you chose to pray, 'Lord, bring my husband home,' be sure you want it answered!"

What I requested of Marty was to visit Miss Mary. When she had a few minutes, if she could stop by and check on her. And she did. Of course, Marty helped in other significant ways, too. I remember one Saturday night when we were invited to a friend's house for a dinner party. By this time, my mother had moved out of her house, and the lawyers wanted all of her silver boxed and stored so that it would not be stolen. I had been out of town with work and had not gotten it done. An hour before the party, we drove to Miss Mary's house. Before us in the dining room was the glass-front credenza jammed with an abundance of silver, pewter and crystal prizes won from a lifetime of bridge and golf tournaments.

There was no time to waste with feelings of being overwhelmed. There was no time to change clothes. And there was no time to go shopping for bubble wrap and packaging tape to protect each piece. Holding in her hand a bottle apparently from *I Dream of Jeannie,* Marty asked, "Keith, where is Mary's collection of tea towels?" I raided the tea towel drawer and for good measure, pillaged the apron drawer, too. I opened another cupboard, and it was chocked full of fabric flour sacks and cloth calendars that had been dutifully recycled into kitchen towels circa World War I. I stacked 'em high on the dining room table, and at a glance, you would have thought that Miss Mary and Aunt Clara did nothing but cross-stitch hand towels.

We began wrapping every silver bowl, tray and pitcher. I packed six boxes full of silver, including an enormous loving cup that Miss Mary won at the Ladies' Golf Classic USA held in Washington, D.C. Magically, seventy-five years of tea towels were about how many we needed. We stored the boxes, reported it "done" to the lawyer, washed and dried our hands using a remaining tea towel with images of giant blueberries and headed out the door to dinner. But according to the old adage, *no good deed goes unpunished.* Apparently, it was time for my punishment. So instead of being thanked for taking care of the silver, I was accused of stealing Miss Mary's silver flatware. Me of all people; I care exactly nothing about eating with an ornate sterling silver fork. The profound truth of Alzheimer's caregiving: every day's experience is irridiculous.

7
Coping Mechanism

The medical school textbook titled *Alzheimer's Disease and Other Dementias* states there are five coping strategies[*] widely used by caregivers that have been identified in clinical settings and research. The coping strategies observed and assessed include:

1) Avoidance
2) Wishful Thinking
3) Blame
4) Problem-Focused Coping
5) Social Support Coping

But there is no mention about what to expect when all five of these coping strategies are used by different children and, in essence, dumped into a Vitamix blender. Push pulse

---

[*] Myron F. Weiner, M.D., and Anne M. Lipton, M.D., Ph.D., eds. *Textbook of Alzheimer Disease and Other Dementias.* Arlington, VA: American Psychiatric Publishing, 2009, 357–358.

a few times. Add some ice. More loud whirring. Watch the swirl. Voila—a foul greasy mess is on your hands that by all accounts looks and smells like a Shit Shake of Family Dynamics. The med-school textbook continues that if you add psychiatric issues that correspond to mood, depression, anxiety, somato-form conditions and alcohol/drug use, the Shit Shake can be turned into an even nastier and more toxic concoction. I guess our researcher and author has observed a percentage of caregivers who were in a generally good mood about Alzheimer's dementia. Sounds to me like 2) Wishful Thinking.

In the never-ending swirl of family dynamics, my clever sister employed this coping option 2) Wishful Thinking and coupled it with 1) Avoidance. Her first step was to stop answering her cell phone altogether. The second step was to leave the phone's voice mailbox full without room for another message. For my mother's nurses and care team, their clinical protocol required contacting the next person— me at work. By successfully avoiding actually talking to a medical professional about an issue, my sister could then employ her Wishful Thinking strategy. And once Libby's Smoke Machine got cranked up, those pesky crazy problems just faded to grey. And if you continued to avoid answering your phone for years, you might be able to feel in control and that dementia really isn't that unpleasant. With this approach, the great hope is that you can keep winning the game of Dodge Ball forever.

By living five hundred miles away and returning home about a day a year, my older brother skipped senior caregiving all together for our father, Great Aunt Clara and Miss Mary. Who could blame him? Why would anyone want to change a Depends diaper on Mary or Bill? The job stinks and does nothing to improve your resume. In fact, in the history of corporate America, no recruiter conducting an interview has ever inquired, "Please tell me about a time when you helped your mom and dad." And for good reason—a caregiver could not tell the truth about helping his mom with Alzheimer's and expect to get the new day job. But when ol' Alzheimer's kicked into high gear, the executive with a masters in accounting and finance was also an experienced master of coping strategy 3: The Blame Game. As the out-of-town expert, he could judge and blame someone else for most any problem erupting out of Alzheimer's mouth. The rules of the game are simple: the problem with me is you. Blame your mother for resisting her care plan. Blame the disease itself. Blame the case worker for not getting it right. Home health care nursing aides and assisted living social workers are sitting ducks. And if you really want to win The Blame Game, you can focus on manipulating the sibling dynamics so that it's two versus one and collectively rise up against your brother. It's the Cain and Abel caregiving strategy for Mom.

Options one through three above may address your issues with Alzheimer's, but they fail to take care of the patient's issues with Alzheimer's. Because the patient requires help, someone must do option 4) Problem-Focused Coping and address the patient's actual health care needs. That would become my job. It seemed reasonable since I had worked in health care for years, was trained to focus on the patient and had helped develop clinical programs to manage chronic conditions. I worked daily with doctors and clinicians in disease management at a high-technology laboratory focused on early identification and treatment of disease. That said, if my sister and brother and I were each going to choose what we were naturally good at, 5) Social Support Coping sounded right for me. I figured it meant drinking beer and bar talk with DougE; kayaking with Dr. Dave, my good friend and neurologist; bonding with Marty about her own parent suffering from dementia. And with my Yogi wife, I assumed Social Support covered sexual-release coping strategies as well.

At times, it felt like I was playing a game of Crazy Eights. The cards had been shuffled and dealt. Each of Miss Mary's children had their own hand and strategies to deal with the matriarch's horrendous death sentence. But as I read and reread chapter 20 about "Family Caregivers," "Caregiver Burden," and "Evidence-Based Interventions," I could find no discussion of money.* I learned that the REACH (Resources for Enhancing Alzheimer's Caregiving Health) study in 2006 had determined that it was cheaper to keep your mom at home rather than pay the bills for a luxury retirement community. Science proved that it's OK to be cheap. I checked the index but neither "money" nor "finances" appeared. I kept looking for the section on caregiving burden about money, control of money, insurance, Medicare/Medicaid, bankruptcy, legal financial reporting, issues of inheritance and the burden that can continue beyond the death of the patient. No guidance. Pussycat, make my Shit Shake a double.

* * *

Senior health care is expensive, and no matter how much you spend on your loved one, money can't cure Alzheimer's. In 2014, the average cost of assisted living in Virginia exceeded $5,000 per month. In Richmond, the range was generally $6,000 to $8,000 per month depending on medical needs. Home health care can be equally costly. And my

---

* Myron F. Weiner, M.D., and Anne M. Lipton, M.D., Ph.D., eds. *Textbook of Alzheimer Disease and Other Dementias.* Arlington, VA: American Psychiatric Publishing, 2009, 353–366.

mother's entire input on her personal finances was: "We don't talk about money."

She was raised to not talk about it, as if money were obscene. My parents didn't cuss, they didn't talk trash about people and they didn't talk about money. I do all of those things and write stories about them, too. But for the Greatest Generation, if you can't say something nice, then don't say anything.

Martha Poppins had expertly advised that Miss Mary could no longer recall financial detail. She said that Miss Mary and I should start piecing together my mom's financial puzzle by collecting all paperwork from every desk drawer and file cabinet in the house and putting it in one place. Little did anyone realize that the boxes, bags and port-a-files would form a mountain of paperwork in my home office. Stock certificates were kept in the long-ago retired briefcase that my father once carried to the office. Terrifyingly, it seemed every canceled check from the past fifty years had been saved. Every statement. Every official-looking letter. As Mary's caseworker informed, it was necessary to look at every piece of paper before throwing it out. The work would take months and generate seven leaf bags of paper to be taken to the shredder.

As I sifted through the mountain of paperwork, the caseworker and lawyer said that it would be important to collect, organize, review and report the finances. There are so many questions about money when a senior has Alzheimer's disease, annual financial reporting is strongly suggested to protect them and their caregiver. As I put all of Mary's finances into a single spreadsheet for the first time in life, it became apparent that Miss Mary wanted exactly no reporting, and her oldest son wanted vastly more reporting. My brother said that he wanted me to send him all information about her finances and estate every three months. My mother was not to pay me for the work. Simultaneously, my mother told me not to send him a thing. Miss Mary wanted total privacy, and he wanted total transparency to the penny. In his mind, they were his pennies. It was no longer clear who had the mental health issues. Lawyer Paul Izzo (and singer Cindy Lauper) got it right: money changes everything. And so does Alzheimer's.

To begin the process, I looked for some sort of financial reporting guidelines from the Alzheimer's Association and other medical and financial organizations. With the prevalence of Alzheimer's in the United States, my problem was nothing new. I assumed there would be guidelines just a Google-search away. But I was wrong. The only standards I could find were from the local County Commissioner of Accounts. A sobering find—these were the accounting guidelines used to review a person's finances after death. They were established out of absolute necessity by lawyers, accountants and investors to resolve family feuds to settle estates.

Mary and Bill—and most from their generation who lived through the Great Depression—put no trust in a single financial institution. They knew from experience that Wall Street and banks can fail you. Money and finances were spread out for a feeling of safety. Mary and Bill had money squirreled away in every tree in the forest. As I looked at each piece of financial paperwork as instructed, hundreds of thousands of dollars in hidden accounts turned up. Mary and Bill took care of themselves. It also explained why we had multiple George Foreman Grills perfectly preserved in the original boxes—once the prize for opening a new bank account.

Martha advised that cash is typically located within a ten-foot radius of a senior's favorite chair or bed. And there it was: cash under the mattress, cash under a chair cushion, cash in a drawer, cash in an old pocketbook. The little old lady was loaded in the house and in the banks. The only thing I found in larger supply were postage stamps of every type, perfectly preserved in No. 6 white envelopes. And we would need those stamps in the upcoming months.

The good part about Mary's finances was that she had scrimped for a lifetime and saved a small fortune. The bad part was that her financial papers were a total mess. The lawyer observed that seniors often seem to be hiding money rather than investing money. Although the PIA (pain in the ass) factor can be high for the family trying to locate and organize finances, the real issue occurs when a senior with Alzheimer's have their savings stolen—and it happens every day. Cases of theft are particularly high with home health care.

* * *

If you're like me, your siblings will let you change all the lightbulbs and Depends you want, but the minute you sign a check, the game has changed. Only the power of attorney has control of the money, and not everyone is happy about it. That's why lawyers are called. Miss Mary needed three things from her lawyer:

1) Power of Attorney
2) Medical Directive
3) Will

But the truth is, there was a number four, the most important one of all:

4) Communication

Without a will, savings may go to Uncle Sam, but it won't make a dent in the national debt. When Aunt Clara was delirious in the hospital, I learned that without power of attorney, no one will be able to make decisions for the patient in the hour of need: financial, legal or medical. Without medical directive, a person can be connected to a feeding tube in a vegetative state for years on end and drive your family into bankruptcy. I also learned the hard way that if a person has not communicated the basic content of these documents and where they are located to the people close to them, it is the same as not having paid lawyers to produce them. My next-door neighbor, Trudy, provided me with a heartbreaking example.

Trudy was reclusive. In her eighties and born in Europe, she had little to do with the neighborhood. A year would pass, and I would see her only a few times, maybe only on Halloween when the kids went to her door trick-or-treating. As she aged, she needed more assistance, and then her husband died of cancer. Every now and then she would ask my wife to pick up a few things from the grocery store or my son to pick up the newspaper. No one else came by her house.

We realized that like many seniors, she had dementia. At the time of her medical emergency, she was not able to call for help. Sadly, she died at home from a fall. Unintentionally, her death set off a series of events that would take months to resolve. The police searched for family and finally located two nephews in upstate New York. John and Joe loaded up the truck with their dogs and headed south to figure out what to do with their estranged Aunt Trudy's estate. After hours of labor—cleaning out old food in the refrigerator, going through boxes of business papers, sorting mail, searching file cabinets— they could find no will. They continued meeting with lawyers, lining up a cleaning service, going through papers and drawers of family photos, washing and waxing her two white Mercedes-Benzes.

And then in a drawer in the living room underneath letters and newspaper clippings, they found a will. Trudy left all of her considerable estate to charity—VCU Massey Cancer Center and others, nothing to family or friends. The only person who could manage the estate was her lawyer. The nephews were in a state of shock. In her heart, she had said goodbye to her family years ago and retreated within herself and her house.

With Mary and Clara, things were far less dramatic. The lawyer came to the house to review their legal documents. The wills were put in order, and the originals stored in the safe deposit box. Aunt Clara was wise and divided her money between charity, nieces and nephews. With a stroke of her pen, she eliminated Bob, her nephew, from the will for "no lack of affection, but he has been paid in full during my lifetime." Mary made only a few tweaks to her will, and then Florence, her loyal friend and housekeeper of thirty years, witnessed as she and Clara signed page after page. The logistics were managed efficiently; the family relationships were not so tidy.

8
Disorganized Religion

As life would have it, Aunt Clara was a caregiver, too. In her seventies before she came to live with my parents, she took care of Aunt Kate. Good-humored Kate was the sole female executive in the finance department of a national insurance company. She liked to brag that she retired early from her finance and accounting career; that is, on her very last day at the office, she left at 4:45, fifteen minutes before closing. About fifteen years after retirement, Kate was diagnosed with "senile dementia," likely Alzheimer's disease. Clara did it all for Kate: the day-to-day care, the doctor appointments, the housework, the bills. She had the type of dementia that we all hope for where you are happy and delusional until the very end of life.

When I asked Aunt Clara how she coped with caring for Kate, she responded, "Me. Oh. My. It was a faith walk. Nothing improves your prayer life like caring for someone with Alzheimer's. Katie kept repeating the same joke endlessly about a boy being spanked on the behind for misbehaving. Sent to his room, he pulled down his pants to inspect the damage. Looking in the mirror he declared, 'Just as I suspected. Split wide open.' Every time, Kate laughed at the punch line like it was the funniest joke that she had heard in life." Clara shared that she didn't think it was very helpful to ask "why" does God allow a terminal disease (or bad joke hell). There aren't a lot of good answers to that one. Rather, the important question is "where" is God in the midst of caring for a person with a disease like Alzheimer's. God is with you, in your heart. Aunt Clara's coping mechanism was a "religious coping strategy" as defined in the medical school textbook on dementia. Saint Clara laughed and agreed wholeheartedly with the textbook description of her coping mechanism and recommended that I read and think about the Gospel of John 19:25-30. I told her I would and looked up John 19 on The Family iPad:

> Now standing beside Jesus' cross were his mother, his mother's sister, Mary the wife of Clopas, and Mary Magdalene. So when Jesus saw his mother and the disciple whom he loved standing there, he said to his mother, "Woman, look, here is your son!" He then said to his disciple, "Look, here is your mother!" From that very time the disciple took her into his own home. ...Jesus said, "It is completed!" Then he bowed his head and gave up his spirit.

So in this pivotal moment of world history, just before Jesus Christ died on the cross to atone for all of mankind's sin… he took time out to care for his mom. Really? "Time Out for Mom" or "Mother Mary to Age with Grace" are not Bible stories I've heard recounted. In a lifetime of sermons, I have not heard the one about the importance of senior care-giving preached by the high priests on Easter or any other Sunday. So which of his siblings did Jesus pick for this job opportunity? Apparently, the Son of God skipped right over Mary's other children and her closest sister in favor of his buddy. John—with his own aging parents—was to become Mary's provider, too, and take her into his own home and help her for the rest of life. On the spot, this fisherman, dis-ciple and teacher was assigned the new role of caregiver. And at the time of his death, Jesus was flat broke and homeless. The King of The Jews had no riches, no palace, no posses-sions, no estate and no physician for the royal family. There was no life insurance or long-term care policy or government Medicare or any financial assistance to pay Mary's way. Talk about dynamics. Apparently "senior health care" has never come with a plan that's easy, cheap or fair.

It's understandable that this story of caregiving for mother Mary has slipped through the cracks of history and has been overshadowed by the other major events of the day. But it did make me wonder, *how did John feel about it?* Was he really Jesus' closest friend as oft reported and prepared to help out? Or was this more like a scene from a Mel Brooks movie, and John happened to be the one standing just a little too close to the foot of the cross when Jesus managed to open an eyelid and see him standing there. The disciple's response to Jesus' directive*: "Who me? Take care of your mother? Forever? Isn't there someone else? After all, this may not be the best use of my gifts…"*

No matter how the details of the story went down, the Son of God's final instruction on Earth was to take care of your mother. An inconvenient point lost in church his-tory. For John, I wonder if senior caregiving was a sacred call that his heart responded to in an ah-ha moment? Or was it more like answering the call on your cell phone from the emergency room in an uh-oh moment? Either way, the swirl of senior caregiving usually begins in an unexpected turn of events and continues winding up an unfamiliar incline. The reward for the caregiving journey must await you in heaven with Mary, Jesus and adopted-son John. The job is too low-profile, too low-paying, too low-thanks and far too contentious for any feel-good reward here on Earth.

About the closest thing I have come across to a sermon on senior caregiving was a media story about Mother Theresa. When this five-foot-tall saint of God was speaking to a large audience of affluent American Christians, she encouraged them not to come to Calcutta on their church's summer mission trip. That's right. She wanted them to stay away from her dirt-poor slum and to stay put in their fertilized fescue-lawn suburb. "We must always remember what God tells us in Scripture: '…I will never forget you.' I want you to find the needy here, right in your own home first. And begin love there. Be that good news to your own family first. And find out about your next-door neighbors. Do you know who they are?"

Mother Theresa called us to remember to take care of the sick, dying and poor who are close at hand. There is no end to the need in the United States with millions of seniors who are sick and dying and blowing their lifetime of savings on health care for Alzheimer's dementia. Like lost sheep, each has gone astray within the darkening landscape of their own mind. Begin love there.

The story of Good Friday continues that once Jesus had died on the cross, "Darkness came over the whole land because the sun's light failed." (Gospel of Luke 23:44,45) In Virginia's own dark times, this is a line of the story that generations of slaves knew by heart who spent their days of endless toil growing tobacco by the banks of the James River. The haunting spiritual the slaves sang about the crucifixion asked, "Were you there when the sun refused to shine?" Like their response, mine is, "Yes, I am there." I know suffering and slow death. I know darkness. With cruel Alzheimer's disease, my understanding of light comes by experiencing darkness. The two are inseparably connected in life. I know light, in part, by its absence. I know God, in part, by his absence. I know love, in part, by its absence.

* * *

For a far less arduous journey than scaling Mount Oldzheimerz, James and I packed what we needed for a weekend hike to Spy Rock. Under a beautiful blue sky, we hiked with Scouts Troop 418 up the side of a mountain in the Blue Ridge to Spy Rock, where Confederate soldiers once spied on encroaching Union Troops. The mountain-top experience was unforgettable with a 360-degree-view of ridges rolling out like blue waves in every direction. The kids climbed the sun bleached granite faces of the summit and explored dark caves for hours.

For dinner, we cooked "hobo packs" of carrots, onions, potatoes with chunks of mystery meat wrapped in aluminum foil over an open fire. In the darkness of night, we huddled there chowing down, telling tales, staying warm. The temperature began dropping. By 10:00 p.m., it had fallen below thirty degrees with a strong north wind. With the campfire burning low and flasks on empty, we moved to our tents. My buddy Richard Moore reached into his stuff sack and pulled out his sleeping bag. Out came a light purple bag with My Little Pony prancing across it, her rainbow mane flowing behind, a treasure belonging to his youngest child, Courtney.

With his North Face sleeping bag stored safely in his attic, My Little Pony was all he had, a SNAFU both hilarious and terrifying. Richard spent that night with half of his body covered by the violet bag and half of his body exposed to the nighttime low of seventeen degrees. Bone cold, shivering and checking his watch every few minutes to see if morning had come, Richard made it through that dark night of the frozen soul. It reminded me of a classic tale about Daniel Boone. He had climbed a tree, up and down and over and over again, to stay warm and survive a frigid Appalachian Mountain night, without even My Little Pony. No one has ever been more thankful for the morning light and warmth of the sun than the stone cold hiker surviving a frigid, dark night on the trail.

Alzheimer's, too, is a close-up study in contrast. The darkness of madness, disease and slow death stands in stark contrast to the good health the person once enjoyed. I knew how demented my mom had become because of how high functioning she had once been. For me, the question became how do I handle the unrelenting darkness? For some people, the answer is to ignore it. For others, the strategy is to plan practical next steps, like installing light sensors to keep track of the wandering Alzheimer's patient at all times. And for others still, darkness consumes them as if they are the one with the disease. For me, I managed with a hybrid of these approaches to caregiving. I stumbled through the unfamiliar and ever-changing landscape as best I could, one misstep at a time.

As darkness came and frigid air blew that night on Spy Rock, my son reached inside his pocket to find his light. He fastened the miner's light with black elastic strap around his head. His headlamp illuminated a small circle about three feet in diameter directly in front of his feet, just enough to keep him moving forward. It provided the light for one next step, and tomorrow's path remained hidden in darkness. Again, I was reminded of caregiving for Alzheimer's dementia. Each day, I had just enough light to navigate one more step through a land where the sun refused to shine. Just enough light that taking the next step required faith to keep truckin' on this long strange trip to journey's end. Just enough light.

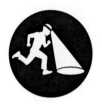

9
Assistance in Living

When Great Aunt Clara was to be discharged from the hospital for the last time, I pulled up www.SeniorLiving.org on my iPad as recommended by the hospital's social worker. The website proclaimed:

> *We'll make selecting the appropriate level of senior care as easy as possible!*

Next to this sunshiny statement was a diagram of a swirling constellation comprised of 15 orange, gold and red spheres each labeled with a senior living arrangement. Starting with the uppermost sphere, the options were:

1) Continuing Care Retirement Center (CCRC)
2) Retirement Community
3) Nursing Home
4) Alzheimer's Care
5) Respite Care
6) Senior Apartment

7) Senior Coop
8) Congregational
9) Assisted Living
10) Hospice Care
11) Personal Care Home
12) Active Senior
13) Independent Living
14) Adult Day Care
15) In-Home Senior Care[*]

When I showed the universe of senior living options to Aunt Clara, she thought she was looking at a cartoon and began laughing. The bubble diagram seemed to her a comedy sketch of a health care cluster fuck, rather than the care options available to her. It was the type of diagram that needed to be accompanied by an expert talking head with a masters degree in health administration to decipher it. After a good laugh, Clara observed, "I don't even see the planet where they want to shuttle me next—'Rehab Facility.' Good heavens, Keith. Drive me home. In life, please do not take me back to this hospital to get fixed again." And that's exactly what she did.

My family's experience is that there are really three primary means of taking care of an aging loved one, with variations of each based on how much professional health care you want to buy:

1) **Family Care** in the home ($)
2) **Home Health Care** with paid professional help ($$)
3) Living at a **Facility for Seniors** with health care by professionals ($$$)

---

[*] "The Senior Living Spectrum." SeniorLiving. 2009. www.seniorliving. org.

Not wanting to miss out (ever), my family did all three. When Aunt Clara was discharged and returned home following the pulmonary crisis, we explored option two and hired a **home health care** service, as she then required a nurse for daily medical care. It is not easy bringing strangers into your house to care for a much-loved family member. The process of interviewing agencies is critical with the main goal of choosing an experienced organization you can trust and a care team that is a fit with your family. Plenty of people warned me against home health care, but I had little choice and no regrets. You can make any care model work, and home health care is effective for many seniors who want to stay in their familiar home environment. We did not experience the horror stories of negligent care, over-billing, theft or scary people showing up at the door. For good measure, I frequently dropped by unannounced to give Aunt Clara a hug and kiss and to check on things. Our family lawyer reviewed and returned the signed contract to the agency and followed-up with a polite call to the director, making his presence known.

Assisted living at a facility for seniors was the best option for my mom when she entered the later stages of Alzheimer's. Twenty-four/seven care was needed with help in all activities: walking, eating, toileting, bathing and communicating. The decision to place mom in such a facility was neither easy nor cheap. But it was the right choice at the right time for Miss Mary, not only for her safety and increasing medical care needs, but also for the social interaction and physical therapy that were critical aspects of her wellbeing.

Providing the right care for an aging person is not a one-and-done decision but rather an on-going process. An Alzheimer's dementia patient's health status does not remain in a fixed position but progresses downhill from stage to stage. And with that change in health status comes ongoing decision making.

Family care is the sole option for more than nine-out-of-ten seniors of the world's population. Think Charlie of Willie Wonka's chocolate factory fame with the entire family living under one roof helping to care for each other. Only in Charlie's case, the elderly enjoyed sleeping together in one ginormous quilt-covered bed. With family care, parents, grandparents, kids and pets live nearby and have a shared generational life, which can be rich in many ways. Most importantly, kids get to know their grandparents, great grandparents and cousins in a deeper and more authentic way. Because you can't get away from these people, you are forced to differentiate and discover who you are as a person in relation to your extended family. Family care is by far the cheapest senior living alternative but also the most draining on resources like time, energy and sanity. I know from first-hand experience. This is the option we chose for my father. He had suffered multiple strokes and Parkinson's disease, among other health issues. We managed his care multiple ways—sometimes doing it all ourselves on the cheap, sometimes using adult day care, sometimes working with Kitty Kat, a favorite LPN who Miss Mary met in the fresh produce section of Ukrop's Super Market.

* * *

As anticipated, Family Care had its ups and downs. I remember being at my home about a mile from my parent's house and watching Super Bowl XXXIV—or at least the first five minutes. The Saint Louis Rams were playing the Tennessee Titans in Atlanta, my wife's hometown. It was the Titans' first appearance at the Super Bowl ever. Evenly matched, either team could win. The Rams' quarterback, Kurt Warner, was on a serious roll. Miraculously, baby

Charlotte was asleep. The chili and cornbread were hot, the beer cold. All was good in America.

The football was snapped, and the game began. As did some sort of interference—not on the field, but in my family room. A loud noise was interrupting the TV sound. *"Is Marty vacuuming ... now?"* My wife attended the University of Virginia, twice—first as an undergraduate and then for graduate school. She held the dubious distinction of never attending a single football game. A product of Georgia, where Jesus and Football are the official state religions, she had exactly zero interest in the game. So not a sports fan, but vacuuming? Housework? Really? *I'll scrub all day tomorrow.*

I listened intently. The noise didn't seem to be coming from inside the house. I went to the window and pulled back the curtain. A precipitation cocktail comprised of sleet, snow, freezing rain and hail—Virginia Winter Mix—was being served up generously. Against the dark purple sky, pellets fell horizontally. A howling Nor'easter was whipping ice directly against the windows on the north side of my house.

I turned back to the TV and watched Kurt Warner snap a perfect spiral, and then the screen went fuzzy. No more reception. The lights flickered. Problems were piling up like snow or cow shit. Then the crack and ensuing chaos of a tree limb falling from the weight of ice. A blackout. No TV. No lights. No furnace. No good.

Marty entered the dark room. "Traveler, can you build a fire? It's going to get cold fast. I put another blanket on the baby. Did your mother make it out?"

Did my mother make it out? The words stopped me cold. My wife was thinking about things other than football, like babies and grandparents and safety. Miss Mary was headed to the airport to catch a plane to Los Angeles to visit her sister, Peggy. I checked my Blackberry, and it was still working. I pulled up Richmond International Airport's flight schedule. Apparently, she boarded the last plane able to fly out of Richmond. As she taxied down the runway and took off for sunny California for a week, the menacing ice storm was right behind her. Miss Mary was out of the storm's reach by a hair, like a Tennessee Titan running full-throttle with the ball and just slipping past the reach of the defensive tackle trying to ground him.

It was good news. These were the days before Alzheimer's was apparent, and she was taking care of both Bill and Clara, and grandbabies were coming fast. She needed a break from the responsibilities of daily caregiving and enjoyed being with her sister. So Miss Mary had left and an ice storm had come, which promoted me to the new interim manager of MAC, the McMullin Advanced Age Center. There were no other applicants.

My cell phone was now dead. The power was out. Winter mix was accumulating, and ice covered the roads. My father, whose health was declining, and Great Aunt Clara were in the same powerless situation, each about a mile from me. I reached for an ice cold beer to celebrate an unforgettable Superbowl Sunday.

In an ice storm, it doesn't matter if you have four-wheel drive, two-wheel drive or front-wheel drive. No wheel is able to gain any traction on ice. With the winter mix coming down, I had no choice but to wait until morning to see my father. At 5:00 a.m., I got out of my sleeping bag by the fireplace, found my L.L.Bean parka and North Face beanie and headed out. I scraped and shoveled for the better part of an hour to uncover my car and driveway under six inches of ice, sleet and snow.

I fishtailed my way to MAC and arrived just in time to watch my father's sitter pull away from the house in her white four-door Ford Fairmont. I watched the back of the car as it slid down the road to freedom. Estelle was out of there.

Because my father required medical care, I had filled out a form and submitted it to the county to bump his address to the top of the list for power restoration. As I entered the split-level house, the lights flickered on, and the oil furnace roared to life. My father and aunt were still sleeping. No need to wake them. It was looking like my pregnant wife, two-year-old daughter and I would be moving into MAC until the spring thaw. Welcome to the wonderful world of Family Care, where there is no home health care agency or assisted living facility to call. It's health care for do-it-yourselfers.

Or perhaps in this case, the daughter-in-law model of health care. Because once four generations were generally taken care of with washing, shaving, changing diapers, clothing, coffee, breakfast and meds—I headed out the door to the office to be able to pay our bills. In health care, the office never closes and our bills need to be paid. Once I left the house, it was my pregnant wife, Marty, on duty. I heard her downstairs wise-cracking with Bill, "If you think I'm going to be giving you your daily sponge bath and hand job, you can forget it. Your girlfriend Kit Kat will be back soon." Words to the wise: if you don't want to wash all of your father-in-law or mother-in-law, start saving for assisted living … beginning now.

Truthfully, most everyone in my family above the age of seventy-five has "assisted living" in one form or another. Miss Mary took care of my father as his health declined. My uncle hired a driver that came four times a week and chauffeured him to lunch, the barber and doctor appointments. An aunt moved in with her daughter and got on the meal plan. A cousin moved into a luxury retirement home. My mother-in-law still lived on the family farm with the help of the farm manager and loyal bookkeeper who lent a hand with yard work, bill paying and errands. Another aunt spent untold thousands to renovate and redecorate a first-floor room into a virtual hospital room complete with electrical upgrade, medical equipment, handicap shower, special toilet and hand rails everywhere.

Horror stories abound about adult kids who do the wrong thing to their parents. The greedy cousin who admitted his kind-hearted father into a cheap and poorly run nursing home to free up money for a trophy wife. The family friend whose father had dementia and whose brother rewrote the father's will leaving the entire estate to himself. He took it all, including college money for grandkids. Our relative whose long-term girlfriend put him in a wheelchair, loaded him on a plane and sent him home so his family could care for him when he was three-quarters dead.

In caring for older parents, I'm surprised by some adult children's complete denial of the What-Goes-Around-Comes-Around principle. Each of us is aging and, in time, will likely need a hand and some assistance with living. Each of us could one day be one of the thirty-five million people worldwide suffering with Alzheimer's. What if each of us is to be assisted exactly as we assisted others?

10
March Madness

Because I lived so close to my relatives, theoretically, I could swing by any evening for a drink. That would include the last week of Aunt Clara's life. As she lay in bed at age ninety-nine with only days remaining of her century-long life, it was easy for me to drop by for one last visit. I was sitting in the swivel chair next to her bed drinking Johnny Walker Black on ice and waiting on death, when my mother said, "Here's the grey box." Over the hospice bed, she passed me a heavy gun-metal grey container, circa 1930, about the size of a safe-deposit box. I asked what was in it, and Miss Mary replied nonchalantly as she headed upstairs to cook dinner, "Her special things, you know. Diamonds."

"Excuse me?"

In the time I knew Aunt Clara, she had never mentioned anything about her Depression-era strongbox. Cold to the touch, the box's weight was significant. As I sat there in the swivel Barcalounger with Aunt Clara gurgling from the fluid filling her lungs, I struggled with the small, slightly bent key to unlock the thing and discover what had been hidden from sight for decades. What exactly would a ninety-nine-year-old, unmarried retired schoolteacher and Saint of God from the hills of eastern Kentucky keep hidden for safe-keeping in this locked treasure chest? I opened the lid, and a stack of United States War Bonds emblazoned with the image of Grover Cleveland spilled to the floor. Land deeds with additional "mineral rights" shrewdly negotiated fell on my lap. Diamond jewelry from long-ago suitors rattled in the bottom under her college diploma and a photograph of her as a 20-year-old heartbreaker. I knew now that it was Clara's choice not to marry. Contracts. Death certificates. Settled estates. Her will with Mary C. McMullin named executor. A postcard from a poetic lover named Ray Schaefer in Colorado. Copies of powerful sermons and devotions. A poem. A Bible verse. A prayer card. An article. More photographs and a century of newspaper clippings of family members that I may or may not recognize.

What did Great Aunt Clara treasure? Faith. Family. Frugality. A well-turned phrase. Fashion, of course. Aunt Clara lived well below her modest means as a schoolteacher and never cashed in the war bonds bought by her father, Caloway. She didn't seem to experience a lack of money or a lack of family or faith. Her niece described her as an independent woman with a heart like King David—a poet's heart—and eyes that see the truth.

After Aunt Clara breathed her last, we began making the arrangements to lay her to rest. The night before the funeral, I was at home watching March Madness on TV. University of Richmond and Virginia Commonwealth University were advancing in the NCAA basketball tournament. My cell phone vibrated. I answered it and headed to the basement, away from the family gathered in my living room. It was Dr. Gergoudis. The time had come to talk. The blue rubber gloves were coming off. "You know, Miss Mary can no longer live alone." The good doctor continued, "Her dementia is progressing. Clara's nurse will need to return to the house to care for her after the funeral and the family leaves."

He patiently explained that Mary should move to something called "Assisted living with continuing care for dementia." The best drugs on the market could not prevent or cure Alzheimer's dementia. What would help my mother the most and provide the highest quality of life possible were exercise programs, a healthy diet, social interaction and feeling safe with twenty-four-hour nurse supervision.

"She should move this month."

It was another bon-a-fide oh-shit moment. I would have done most anything for the good doctor to call a couple weeks after Aunt Clara's funeral and to say something along the lines of *we should begin thinking about moving this year*. But my personal timeline was not on the table for discussion.

Stunned, I responded profoundly. "Uh huh."

With Aunt Clara now gone, Mary would be living alone for the first time in life. She would be entering a period of transition and adjusting to a new normal. Her Alzheimer's disease was moderate, but her health was on the decline. There was no stopping Alzheimer's from advancing. It was no longer safe for Miss Mary to live alone. She could forget and take too many meds. She could forget and leave the stove burning. She could go for a walk and forget the route home. I knew that all of these things had already occurred, and on some days she struggled using stairs and on other days she forgot how to use the phone. In which case, she wouldn't be able to call for help if she needed it.

Dr. Gergoudis explained that Miss Mary did have the ability to manage the transition to assisted living. He felt she could manage this type of major life change one time successfully. But she no longer had the ability or resiliency to manage five, six or seven transitions in care. Living in a new place requires the ability to learn and recall new information, like where the toilet is. Miss Mary, our honor student, was struggling to learn anything new.

Dr. Gergoudis warned that a typical pattern for a senior with increasing care needs could look something like this:

1) Transition to **home health care** during the daytime
2) Transition to the **hospital** for emergency care as a result of a fall or injury
3) Upon discharge from the hospital, transition to a **short-term rehab facility**
4) Upon discharge from rehab, transition back home with **home health care** around the clock
5) Transition to **any assisted living** that is admitting seniors
6) Transition to **assisted living**, the place you prefer with the right level of care.

The doctor continued that this is a common and often harmful course of action. It is more change than any senior could manage, let alone a person with dementia. You can be transitioned to death. Realistically, he advised that we transition Miss Mary to an assisted living facility where she and the family would like her to be. (Translation: skip steps 1 through 5 above.) He encouraged me to make sure we chose a facility that could manage the full spectrum of care for an Alzheimer's patient. It doesn't work well for the senior to be relocated again and again as Alzheimer's progresses. That pattern for a person with dementia looked something like this:

1) Transition to general **assisted living** in the mild stage of Alzheimer's

2) Transition to a new facility and move into **assisted living for dementia** as Alzheimer's progresses to the moderate stage
3) Transition to a new facility with a **"nursing bed"** and full care in the severe stage
4) Transition one last time to **hospice** at end of life.

Dr. Gergoudis suggested looking at continuing care retirement communities that could manage the full continuum of care for Mary until the end of life. He added, "I have known her for a long time. She is a remarkable woman. Her IQ tested at the genius level. It has taken Alzheimer's a long time to diminish her to the point where her mental capabilities are below normal. She is just now getting there."

Dr. Gergoudis knew my mother well. "Once you begin looking at facilities that can provide the care she needs, the list will be reduced to a few. If the care is equivalent, consider the place closest to the family. Mary's greatest fear is that she'll be isolated from her grandchildren."

I've often thought the single most important thing any child can do for an aging parent is to find them a good doctor. That is, a doctor who is well trained, experienced in geriatric care, respected by his colleagues at the admitting hospital and most importantly, patient-focused with a history of strong health outcomes. Dr. Gergoudis concluded our conversation by saying, "Keith, your mother is as proud of her children and grandchildren as y'all are of her. Even with dementia, she is a beautiful and remarkable woman."

So after Clara's memorial service and lunch and a thousand funeral logistics, we ran short of time. Yet again. So Grammy Mary had to come with me to James's piano lesson before I had time to take her home. We sat and talked quietly, listening to him play a song titled *Everything's Ducky.* Once home, we sat in the living room on the white loveseat, and I delivered the first piece of news, "The doctor said nurse Jennifer needs to return tomorrow morning." Mary was shocked with the realization that the nurse was coming for her. "This is the Alzheimer's isn't it?" she asked. I replied, "Yes, it is."

After more conversation, she leveled her gaze at mine and spoke directly, "We will make the best of a bad situation." And like Great Aunt Clara before her, she was a champion to the end.

* * *

Choosing a New Home

How do you choose an assisted living facility for your mother? For me, the first large obstacle to surmount was the name. Would I really move my mom to a place named "Tara?" Would Scarlett, Rhet, Mammy and the gang be there, too? Or would she be happier in "Elysian Fields" with unicorns, sparkly glitter and daffodils in bloom all year? Perhaps "Sunrise" would be better where blackbird has spoken, and the world would be new like the very first morning? Surely no one could go wrong with care-options like these.

Once I became immune to absurd branding, Internet research showed more than a hundred options for senior care within fifteen miles of Miss Mary's house. There was bound to be one that would meet her care needs. Funneling the list down to a handful of facilities was far easier than it first seemed by using a handful of criteria:

1) Miss Mary's primary care physician had diagnosed her with Alzheimer's dementia with complications including vertigo. There was no way to hide it or to get around this diagnosis as the facility's medical director

would review her medical history. Her diagnosis alone reduced the number of places that could provide the care she needed from more than a hundred to fewer than ten.

2) Miss Mary needed a place that could provide the care she would need until the end of life, including hospice care. There was no way my mother could play musical chairs and manage changing facilities and care teams every time her care needs increased. We were down to five facilities.

3) Miss Mary's preference was to live in a faith-based assisted living facility with church services that she could attend. That narrowed the list to three or four.

4) The facility must have an opening for a senior to be admitted directly into assisted living, skipping the first step of "walking in" to independent living. This left two potentials.

5) With care being equal, she wanted to live nearby her family and grandkids. One.

Over the course of the previous year, I had explored several options for either Aunt Clara or my mom. Primarily on my lunch hour, I had looked at numerous retirement homes to get an idea of facilities, space and cost. I now realized I didn't need to look at more than a handful. And with the recommendations from experts like Dr. Gergoudis, caseworker Martha and the hospice nurse, I probably could have looked at just three in one afternoon.

Lakewood Manor was the assisted living facility that opened the door for Miss Mary. They had exactly one room available, and it was exactly the kind she needed. They were no longer admitting directly into assisted living, but since I had met with them the previous year, a grandfather clause ushered us in. My mother could move as soon as a pile of paperwork and evaluations were completed. It looked like she was moving to the Best Exotic Marigold Hotel in India, not to assisted living a couple miles down Patterson Avenue.

With health care, red tape is a given. Martha Poppins helped me, and truthfully, I really didn't mind the paperwork because if Lakewood didn't work out, I didn't have a good option number two. My mother's trusted physician, Dr. Gergoudis, would remain her doctor at the facility. Mary had a second checking account, one to which she deposited the government's money (a.k.a. Social Security checks) to return to the government when it was time to pay their taxes. Over the years, that checking account had accrued enough to cover the Lakewood Manor's entrance fee without touching her savings, critical for Miss Mary's agreement to the deal. Lakewood's social worker and accountant had experience working with Mary's long-term care insurance company. And the icing on the nursing home cake was that Mrs. Sparks, mom's former neighbor, was moving into the same suite.

The first time I took Mary to look at Lakewood, she was polite to Nona, the administrator, and Gladys, the nurse. We toured and talked. As we were walking to the exit, mom cut her eyes toward me and said, "Nothing but a well-decorated prison." I howled laughing at the surprise attack and suggested we tour a cinderblock Medicaid facility I knew downtown. We talked more, and she revealed that when she was about twenty, she worked in a mental institution in Lexington, Kentucky. Essentially it was run like a prison, and she had a deep-seated fear of being institutionalized. I could not ease her fear, but her caseworker could. Miss Mary listened to Martha, a respected subject-matter-expert.

Miss Mary consented to come back for an interview. Thankfully, she looked her best and dialed up the Southern charm. She talked about her family and her friends who lived there. Lakewood is a Baptist facility, so she shared her experience of being one of the first women faculty at University of Richmond, a Baptist-founded college. Dr. Gergoudis was our reference, and after he spoke with the administrator, Miss Mary was accepted that afternoon.

The monthly cost at Lakewood would range from $6,000 to $8,000, depending on the level of care and medical supplies required. In the final analysis, I was surprised that it really was Uncle Sam who picked up her tab for the care at Lakewood. Although Miss Mary had considerable resources, she was feeding at the government trough. Medicare picked up the lion's share of her medical and pharmaceutical bills. And when she entered hospice, Medicare covered one hundred percent of the medical costs. Miss Mary paid the admission fee for Lakewood from her Social Security checking account. Years ago she had purchased long-term care insurance with Penn Treaty located in Pennsylvania. Her policy included a rider covering care for Alzheimer's disease. Apparently, the company's underwriters failed to accurately estimate the skyrocketing costs of senior health care, and Penn Treaty was in bankruptcy proceedings. While in a "rehabilitation" phase, the State of Pennsylvania was running the show and its tax payers were helping pay for Miss Mary's claims costs. The reality was that good taxpayers would largely foot my mother's monthly bills for Lakewood Manor. Between Social Security, Medicare and the State of Pennsylvania, Miss Mary did not touch her personal savings for the excellent health care she received until her last day. Sure it required the thankless job of filling out forms every month, but that was time well spent considering the millions of seniors in the United States with Alzheimer's dementia in need of quality care.

Even though health care is extremely expensive, the social worker warned that a surprising number of children raid the piggy bank once mom is moved to assisted living. They help themselves to her savings, assuming there is more than enough money to pay the bills or that Medicare/Medicaid should pay anyway. Needless to say, the day comes when there is no longer enough money to pay mom's escalating health care bills, and tough decisions have to be made. Greed is so common, the social worker advised reading our contract carefully to understand if "gifting" would break our agreement with the facility.

While looking at Lakewood Manor and other facilities, I had been concerned about the cost as well as the space. She would have only one private room that would open to a suite and common rooms. I shared my concern with Gladys, the nurse who had worked with seniors for many years. She reassured me, "It really is the right amount of space for your mom at this point in her life." I reminded myself that I had lived in a dorm room and a one-room apartment. In Japan, her accommodations would be considered a palace. Nonetheless, it seemed small, a long way from her four-bedroom house where for fifty years she had accumulated clothes in every closet. In time, Gladys proved to be exactly right. One room, one bathroom, one closet was all the space that Miss Mary could manage. And once she was settled into her new room, the "spells" of vertigo decreased significantly. Miss Mary was getting the right level of care at the right time in the right space.

* * *

The Crowbar

When I told Miss Mary's girlfriend we were able to get a room in assisted living at Lakewood Manor, she hugged me with relief. "I feel like she just got in Princeton. With

Alzheimer's, I just wasn't sure where Miss Mary could go. You've got to be able to "walk in" on your own to be admitted to assisted living. Only your mother could pull this one off." And then she summed up our next predicament, "I can't imagine the size of the crowbar you'll need to pry Mary out of her house, kicking and screaming. Call her doctor and make an appointment to let him give her the big first shove. Don't you worry, Richard Gergoudis is an old pro. I'll drop by for a visit and give her another nudge."

And so the nudging began to pry her loose. Some key phrases:

1) The Doctor said …
2) Dad always said …
3) You planned for this …
4) It is a privilege to live at Lakewood Manor …

Dr. Gergoudis did give the first big push to dislodge her from her home where she raised three kids and lived with her husband and aunt. The doctor spoke plainly about his own parents and the poor decisions his family had made about their care. He talked about their declining health and how they struggled to get appropriate care when needed. He wholeheartedly endorsed Lakewood Manor and said that he wished his parents could live there. Mary listened.

We had saved the "Bill" trump card for years, and my wife played it expertly. She arranged a "ladies' luncheon" with Miss Mary and shared the story that Bill had instructed me before he died to "take care of your mother." I had agreed. Marty shared about her father, Ole Daddy. "There comes a point when it is no longer safe or a good idea to live alone. Like with the three flights of stairs in your house, it's so easy to slip. Alzheimer's doesn't make anything easier."

"Oh, yes."

She reminded her that Bill, an engineer in research and development, expected us to make good and reasonable decisions, like taking advantage of the services provided by Lakewood. Miss Mary respected Bill's opinion, even seven years after his death.

What sealed the deal was the long-term care insurance that she had bought in her fifties. She heard a speaker on the subject and thought it sounded like a good idea. At the time, her own mother was dying of Alzheimer's, and she understood and feared the disease. At some level, she was making plans to live in assisted living one day. Incredibly, she sent in her $46 check every month and never missed a payment. A lawyer's dream, Mary saved every piece of paperwork. Over the years, she bought a rider covering Alzheimer's disease, one providing an annual standard of living increase and a rider covering her until end-of-life. She was also a caregiving son's dream. Far from easy, it can be a significant challenge to meet all the criteria necessary for a long-term care insurance company to pay a claim. However, Miss Mary had what she needed to successfully process her claims: perfect documentation, a doctor and lawyer on her side, a case worker who understood the system and a son who would fill out every irridiculous form thrown at him. They covered her in full.

Of the many perspectives on assisted living—medical, family, financial—perhaps the most important is from 30,000 feet high. Living at Lakewood Manor Assisted Living is a privilege. Of the world's population, about one percent of seniors are able to live at a place like Lakewood and receive high-quality care until the end-of-life, no matter what type or how much care they need.* Rather than a

---

* Prof Martin Prince et al., "An Analysis of Prevalence, Incidence, Cost & Trends." *World Alzheimer Report: The Global Impact of Dementia*, Alzheimer's Disease International, September 2015.

death sentence or something that must be endured, assisted living is for the privileged few. Alzheimer's is a cruel disease. To be given quality medical care is something of a miracle.

* * *

The Transition

It would be no small challenge to get Miss Mary and her belongings physically moved from her house to Lakewood Manor. Caseworker Martha advised us that it was not possible for a senior with Alzheimer's to manage a move on her own. Her brain no longer had the capability and executive decision-making function needed to make the hundreds of decisions required in the process of downsizing and moving. In addition, neurologist Dr. Dave shared that she was likely experiencing apraxia. That is, her brain no longer had good communication with her muscles. At times her hands quivered and her feet shuffled. She could not effortlessly fold and pack clothes and tote a box like she once could. On the day of her move, all that should be expected of Miss Mary was to wake up, get dressed, be chauffeured to Lakewood and arrive in style at her new room magically decorated with her favorite things. Her high-energy granddaughter, Charlotte, would give her a tour of her room and show her where everything was kept. Martha Poppins referred to the move as The Transition. She explained that with dementia, it was mission-critical for the move to go smoothly to help with this major change to a new environment.

She recommended a professional moving company called Door-To-Door Solutions, a company with specialized health care knowledge and expertise in moving seniors with dementia from their home into assisted living. She felt it would make the move easier on everyone involved. I was in need of something being easier. I contacted the company and was told they could manage the entire move with the exception of two personal items that were the responsibility of the family: clothes and pictures. When Lakewood Manor asked us directly who would be managing clothes, my sister, the stay-at-home-diva, raised her hand and accidentally joined The Transition Team. Yet another oh-shit moment. Soon after, Lakewood's staff delivered the news that the move-in date which worked for their facilities team and the moving company was Libby's birthday, apparently interfering with spa plans. What was The Transition Team thinking? This outrageous decision was too much to endure quietly and led directly to Meltdown 2009, featuring dramatic angry screaming. Apparently, there was more at stake here than which red turtleneck to pack.

The fact of the matter was that there were far fewer dynamics at play when your style-less son in khaki pants stated, "Mom, there is room for one Christmas sweater. Not one hundred. Which is it going to be—jingle bell Rudolph or sparkle Christmas tree? Which is your favorite, Grammy?"

"Sparkle."

"Perfect."

The only thing that possibly could be more ridiculous than an argument over "sparkle sweater," would be an argument over a Christmas apron. None would be packed for Lakewood. The room had no kitchenette, and there was no use for an apron. No exceptions. In her crafty way, my wife eased Grammy's anxiety by recycling designer aprons circa 1950 into a skirt covering the base of our Christmas tree, a lasting tribute to Miss Mary. Whatever it takes.

Martha Poppins advised us to keep it simple. We were moving from a four-bedroom house to a one-room apartment of sorts. For a senior with dementia, it would be very important to move her most familiar things. Martha told us to move the bed she slept in, the blankets she used, the nightstand and clock kept by that bed, the dresser regularly used with its drawer contents about the same and the chair where she read the newspaper and watched TV. Then add a few small things to her new space: a table, a bookcase, a favorite lamp. When a well-intentioned family member goes shopping and buys all new furniture so that the senior will have a beautifully appointed room, it can backfire. The senior can become disoriented and struggle to recall where her belongings are. The Transition to assisted living is made considerably more difficult and lengthy. Miss Mary's new room should look and feel like her home, her familiar nest.

Martha suggested that we give her a month for The Transition. This was a major life change, and it would take some time to adjust. "Give her a while to settle and to make new friends," I remember her wisely telling me. "Ask her questions other than, 'How did you like it today?' Similar to when a gardener transplants a flower, he can't pull it out of the ground every day and check on the roots to make sure they are doing OK. Your mother will establish a new pattern with meals, activities and meds and will adjust to her new life."

* * *

More Tending

To help with The Transition, Martha suggested that I spend the night with mom at her house before she moved to Lakewood. She said it was a good idea to have a family member with her on Tuesday night in case she experienced confusion or anxiety about so much change. Miss Mary's immediate response to the idea was, "Why in the world would you spend the night with me in the middle of the week? Don't you have a job and family to tend to?"

"Thank you for remembering. In fact, I have an early morning meeting on Wednesday that I do need to tend to. Tuesday evening, I'll cook dinner, and we'll hang out and watch *The Andy Griffith Show* or *Murder She Wrote* on TVLand. Wednesday, I'll get up early for a 7:30 meeting downtown and be back here by 9:00 to drive to Lakewood."

"All right, Darlin'. While you're gone to your meeting, I'll get ready for the day. Do you remember Elsie Sparks? She will be my new neighbor."

"Sounds good."

When the time came for the sleep-over, I found myself wondering why I was doing so much packing of my own clothes when Miss Mary was the one moving. I came rushing from the office loaded down like a Sherpa with my own baggage. Today's sport coat. A duffle bag with jeans and polo shirt for Tuesday night. Hangers with Wednesday's clothes for the office. The gym bag. My briefcase and computer. The shaving kit. As I trudged up Miss Mary's stairs carrying my burdens, I instinctively headed to my old bedroom as a kid. But that seemed weird—it was Aunt Clara's bed that she had slept in until death. I turned to the guest bedroom with my grandmother's double bed (the bed she had died in), but it had been turned into a staging area and was covered with vibrant-colored stacks of sweaters and dresses purchased at decades of super sales. We had raided the furniture in the third bedroom for use at Lakewood, but there remained a mattress on the floor from an old trundle bed. *Any port in a storm,* I thought to myself and laid my stuff at the foot of the mattress.

Tuesday night was Taco Night, and that was exactly what I was capable of cooking. It would be a different child who prepared a five-course final meal and served it on the wedding china with crystal wine goblets. I grabbed the familiar Mexene Chili Powder jar—"The Chili Champion's

Choice"—with its blue lid and foil label from the wood spice rack made in eighth-grade shop class. I reached my hand into the red net bag and found my mother's very last yellow onion. I began chopping with a knife that had not been sharpened in years. The familiar handle was made of deer antler, and apparently, the knife had been handed down from Caveman McMullin. I felt a tear beginning to run down my cheek. If the onion got me crying, it also got me thinking—just how much were we, the caregivers, expecting Miss Mary to give up during the next twenty-four hours? Just how much were we expecting her to lose and to be pleasant about the loss?

She had already lost her husband and life partner and was no longer "wife." She had just lost Aunt Clara, the last of a generation, and was no longer "niece" or "caregiver." She was giving up her house of fifty years and was no longer "owner." She was giving up housekeeping. She was giving up cooking and gardening and the daffodils she transplanted from her great-grandmother's yard. She was giving up her neighborhood and living independently in her community. She was giving up a fashion mound of outfits collected over a lifetime. She had already given up driving and was even declined a parking spot for The GramCam at Lakewood. It must be jettisoned, too.

I passed her the slotted spoon to brown the onion in the black cast-iron skillet. She added the ground beef; it would be the last time that I would hear the sound of her World War II military-issue spoon clicking against the iron skillet as the red meat sizzled and turned brown. The industrial-style exhaust fan installed by my father in 1970 was sucking every fume out of the house. Matter-of-factly, Grammy Mary commented, "I no longer can smell or taste much... and my eyesight isn't much better. You add the Mexene's and make it as hot as you like. There is nothing worse than having an empty stomach and the food's too hot to enjoy." She had not yet lost all her marbles. Over dinner, she informed me plainly, "The time has come for me to move from my home. I'm leaving a lot for you to clean up behind me. I'm sorry about that, Keith. I just can't manage everything like I once did. But there is one thing I am not prepared to be without. That is my grandchildren." Of all the roles and all the activities we were asking her to give up in a twenty-four-hour window of time, Miss Mary drew the line at "grandmother." That was a title not even Alzheimer's would manage to strip from her.

The time had come for me to lay it on the line. "Mom, a house can be taken away. A car and three or four sofas can be taken away. You can take away cooking and cleaning. Thank, God. But no one can take away your grandchildren and the love and respect they feel for you. Charlotte is coming to see you tomorrow at Lakewood after school. She has a surprise she wants to give you."

"Well, this is certainly a week of surprises. Please tell Charlotte that I'll be expecting her."

* * *

More Kayaking

Once Miss Mary was moved, I headed to the bar and Doug bought me a couple beers. We joked, and I asked our time-honored question: *Where is the finish line?* Although my mom was moved to assisted living, the work was nowhere near over. Using the Kayak Method, I did one thing a day for her. I kept a log of the daily phone calls I made on her behalf, many just to change her address or disconnect a service. After a month, I accumulated the following list:

- doctor
- bank (new checks)
- lawyer
- accountant
- post office
- credit card
- water/sewage
- electrical
- oil for furnace
- lawn
- housekeeper
- trash
- homeowner insurance (which became renters' insurance)
- health insurance
- Medicare
- cable (reconnect)
- phone (reconnect)
- voter registration
- church
- charities
- IRS
- Social Security
- financial companies/investments/pension
- newspaper
- magazines
- car (DMV, insurance, Smart Tag, AAA)
- memberships
- clubs, associations
- www.donotcall.gov

With each phone call, each "oar" in the water, we reached our destination within a few weeks. The only rock that unapologetically smashed into the kayak was the telephone company. Their customer service rep based in India had my eighty-two-year-old mother, with Alzheimer's dementia, using a borrowed cell phone and on all fours behind her recliner trying to adjust the phone jack herself. Because the phone company is so unbelievably difficult and beyond reason, I knew to expect nothing else. In fact, the little old ladies at Lakewood Manor collectively filed a complaint against them. Miss Mary's 92-year-old neighbor had a different approach in mind—she politely requested that I have a bomb dropped on their headquarters to send Verizon to the horizon. Another day's kayak stroke.

* * *

With Miss Mary now comfortably settled at Lakewood Manor, it was time to begin dispersing her belongings and getting the house ready to sell. That, of course, would involve lawyers. I worked on emptying the house and ensuring that each child received what was earmarked for them in Miss Mary's will. Always contentious, my out-of-town brother and my in-town sister sent threatening emails and declared they were not comfortable with putting a "For Sale" sign in the front yard. My brother was, however, comfortable with a promotional flier that, once approved by him, I could print and hand out myself. I got a good laugh about the proposed game of "Brother may I... pretty please with a cherry on top." As fate would have it, while I was cleaning out the shed, a couple pulled into the driveway and asked about the house. I gave them a tour and answered questions about the roof shingles, HVAC system and the termite exterminator we had used for decades. They made a cash offer.

During this time, Grammy Mary invited our family to join her for dinner at Lakewood. While sitting at the table, Miss Mary—the child of the Great Depression—instructed her grandchildren plainly, "Not everyone lives in a luxury

retirement home with gourmet meals. While you are cleaning out my house, take what you want from my kitchen and
give the rest of the food to someone who can use it."

Her nine-year-old grandson, James, took her seriously
word-for-word. At his leading, he, Charlotte and I headed to
her house after Saturday soccer practice. We went through
the corner cupboard in the kitchen and emptied it of white
rice, egg noodles, and multiple boxes of Hamburger Helper
Stroganoff. When your mother has Alzheimer's, there is
never just one of any item. We emptied the cabinet over the
stairs and added multiple cans of Campbell's Tomato Soup
to the bounty. We cleaned out the downstairs closet full of
canned green beans, yams, collard greens, shoe peg corn and
Pocahontas tomatoes. We got the three boxes of marble cake
mix off the top shelf in the utility room. (We threw out Mrs.
Ann Friend's canned watermelon rind pickles, circa 1900.)
The kids saved for themselves Aunt Clara's six-pack of Coca-
Cola in green glass bottles and Duncan Hines double-choc-
olate brownie mix. I had no idea what we should do with a
lifetime supply of Comet cleanser and GE lightbulbs.

Then we raided the collection of perfectly folded brown-
paper bags from Ukrop's Super Market and packed the food
stuffs. Charlotte and James loaded the back of the Highlander
and as good citizens, we took it to my office and filled the
company's donation box to overflowing for the Virginia Food
Bank for those in need. All as Miss Mary intended.

The following Tuesday, I was at the office and generally
swamped saving humanity from various disease states. I was
on the phone with the New York office and looked at my
watch. It was 2:00 p.m., and lunchtime was over before it
had begun. Hungry and late to the next meeting, I left my
office and passed the kitchenette. Outside the door was our
food donation box for Virginia Food Bank. Sitting on top
was the iconic red-and-white can of Campbell's Tomato

Soup my kids donated from Miss Mary's house to feed the needy. I looked around to make sure I was alone, reached in and snagged it. As I was reading "JUST HEAT & ENJOY," Thayer walked around the corner from the team meeting. "Really?" he smirked.

Speechless, my mind raced. *"You have a problem with me stealing fucking food from the homeless? There is a quasi-rational explanation, if you've got the rest of the day. You see, my mother lived in her house for fifty years. And when she moved to assisted living, she asked her grandkids to donate all of the food, including this soup to feed the hungry. That is why I am checking the expiration date and am about to heat and eat this three-year-old soup. I'm someone who can use it..."*

* * *

Later that summer after my mom was successfully transplanted to Lakewood, Hurricane Irene roared through town; its damage was devastating. Two oak trees fell across my neighbor's house. Debris covered cars and roads. Electric and cable lines hung lifeless, and it would take more than a week for order and power to be restored. As the sun was rising in the clear blue sky that follows a hurricane, I walked around my own house and checked for damage. For years, storms meant checking on my mom's property as well. In the past, I would have called DougE and borrowed a generator from his commercial construction company to keep Aunt Clara's medical equipment humming.

I cleared the driveway of branches so that I could drive the Highlander SUV to Lakewood to check on Miss Mary. Downed power lines and electrical poles snapped off by high winds littered the roads. It was slow going and required taking side roads that were not blocked or flooded. As I pulled into Lakewood Manor, the lights were magically on. The automatic doors slid open. It was before seven a.m., and the receptionist was already seated at her desk, calmly answering the phone. I thought I had arrived at Disney Land.

The smiling nurse opened the door when I arrived at Mary's suite. The nurses and aides were all there, ready and in uniform, starting the day like always: waking seniors and managing meds. Mary was in her room putting on makeup and getting ready for another day. Her daily rituals peacefully took place without any interruption from Mother Nature. Someone other than me was managing the backup generator, assisting with the living.

* * *

That summer after Miss Mary's house was sold, I stood on the back patio wrangling her house key off my key ring and handed it to the sassy blonde real estate agent for the new owner. I felt an incredible lightness of being. I was no longer fettered to MAC; the era of property management had ended. No more light bulbs to replace. No more fallen trees to remove. No more driveway drainage issues to resolve. No more handrails to install. No more refrigerator ice machines to repair. After fifteen years of service, I finally set the wheel barrow down. Hands free.

Managing senior health care is one of the most difficult jobs I've had. In addition to house maintenance, every day brings a new challenge, like managing home health care, choosing an assisted living facility, applying and being accepted into an assisted living facility, moving, selling the house, finances, Medicare, family dynamics, memory loss, medication adherence, safety, driving, physical therapy, communication, loss of control… the list goes on. But of all these things, I think the toughest part of caregiving for me is pace and flow. Miss Mary's pace slowed to a fraction of her previous life speed. Words got hung up, especially later in the day. Ideas had to rise to the surface and maybe didn't appear until the next day. Walking slowed and going up stairs nearly ceased. Multi-tasking was out of the question. The high performer became the slow responder. Time no longer held the same meaning and became irrelevant.

I remember one evening when Miss Mary and Aunt Clara were living together, I left the office after back-to-back meetings to swing by their house to complete another form for the Medicare Supplement policy. I needed a couple of details and a signature. I had just a few minutes before it was time to pick up James at soccer practice. As I walked in the door sure that this job would only take a minute, I could feel the Blackberry buzzing in the pocket of my sport coat.

Miss Mary answered the door with a "Hello, Sugar. Won't you have a drink?" We sat on the white love seat in the living room. Miss Mary was ready for cocktail hour. She talked about Peggy coming to visit. Trout fried in the kitchen. The familiar sounds and smells of fish, greens and rice came from the kitchen door. Mary asked about her grandkids. Her agenda was simple—visit with one another. Mine was simple—fill out another government form. The two goals were not aligned. The corporate executive going seventy-files per hour in the far-left lane needed to slow down and pull over on the right shoulder. It was time to try putting into practice two "Ps" that my company CEO, Tom Byrd, persistently preached: 1) Patience and 2) Perspective.

With an Alzheimer's senior, it is not possible to enforce your agenda. You can only work with their agenda at their pace. People who cannot embrace this idea are the ones you see yelling and endlessly correcting the senior in their care. It is painful to watch. The person who stands over their parent and starts every sentence with, "I told you …" It's as if by scolding and correcting, the Alzheimer's senior will suddenly regenerate healthy brain cells and short-term memory will begin functioning. They treat their parent like a misbehaving child who can be corrected rather than a patient whose brain is atrophying. Inside the person with Alzheimer's, the light no longer works in every room. The internal wiring has shorted out. No words, no medications, no treatment is going to fix that light and make it burn brightly again. Sometimes the light may jiggle on for a moment, but that's a gift to receive, not one that's on demand.

In the United States, we are not wired to let go. But the time comes when a senior with dementia can no longer drive, both literally and figuratively, and must let go of the steering wheel. A caregiver must sit in the driver's seat and steer and set direction. Alzheimer's is the master teacher of letting go. My mother had to let go of her mind. Let go of her house and housekeeping. Let go of control. Let go of her person. I had to let go of my agenda. Let go of my time. Let go of things making sense. Let go of my mom.

Dr. Reinhold Niebuhr, professor at Union Theological Seminary, wrote an often-repeated prayer at Red Cross field hospitals for the sick and dying during World War II. It is still oddly relevant for caregivers battling Alzheimer's:

> God grant me the serenity,
> to accept the things I cannot change…
> Courage to change the things I can,
> and the wisdom to know the difference.
> Living one day at a time,
> Enjoying one moment at a time,
> Accepting hardship as a pathway to peace.

Dealing with Alzheimer's is about how you function amidst dysfunction. The daily challenge is looking for clarity, letting go and finding peace. It is worth it in the end. After your loved one has died, you can look yourself in the mirror and say, "I did the best I could functioning in slow-motion disaster."

11
Troublesome Creek

When the day finally arrived to probate Aunt Clara's will, I took an hour off from work and drove Miss Mary in The GramCam to the County Courthouse. After being nearly strip-searched by security (up and to the right, please), we sat and waited on a deacon's bench for the better part of an hour to see the County Clerk and Commissioner of Accounts. In a manila file folder I had Clara's birth certificate, death certificate, obituary, certified will, diagram of numerous nieces and nephews to whom she was leaving money and jewelry and a stack of other papers. No sooner had we sat down with the Commissioner than he said, "Mrs. McMullin, I believe your aunt's lawyer is Paul Izzo with ThompsonMcMullan. Paul is a rare find—a respected lawyer. I have known him for many years, and in fact, I talked with Paul. He spoke highly of Miss Napier. Mrs. McMullin, I need to ask if you have been diagnosed with Alzheimer's dementia. Has Dr. Richard Gergoudis spoken to you about having Alzheimer's disease?"

That morning, Miss Mary's mind was not failing her. She assessed the situation and responded with poise, "Yes. If your concern is that I may not be the right person to serve as executor for my aunt's estate, I concur. My son, Keith, has lent a hand to help Clara and me for years. He will settle the estate."

And yet another oh-shit moment. Miss Mary implemented a pre-meditated Plan B, and I was appointed executor for my Great Aunt's estate. Before I could raise my hand to ask about Plan C, the Commissioner and Clerk stamped documents codifying Plan B. In addition to being husband, father, son, health-care executive, breadwinner and caregiver for a parent with Alzheimer's, I had also been named, "Executor for Clara Ethel Napier." Executor of an estate to benefit about a dozen second cousins, most of whom were retired with damn little to do other than wake up, drink coffee and read obituaries in the morning newspaper. My generation did not benefit from the will, ensuring my inheritance from Aunt Clara would not be money.

For Aunt Clara, like most of us, life came to a close with a yard sale. The burial takes care of your body, but not your stuff. For all eternity, your stuff is sold and sold and sold. Aunt Clara's will made it clear: her jewelry was to be distributed to her nieces, and her other belongings were to be sold. The proceeds would be added to her surprisingly large estate and distributed. On faded paper, her perfect penmanship spelled out the names of nieces and which piece of jewelry she "bequeathed" to them. Great Aunt Clara died at age ninety-nine. Her nieces were not a whole lot younger. Well-adorned Napier descendants would be turning up at Movie Night and Bingo in continuing care retirement centers across the country.

On Saturday after Charlotte's lacrosse practice, she and I drove to Miss Mary's house. Charlotte made a bee-line upstairs to Aunt Clara's room and carried down the jewelry box hidden from the light of day and set it on the dining room table. We had about an hour and thought we could sort the jewelry to help settle the estate. One box came downstairs, then Charlotte came down with another, then another … and still another. Unfortunately, in my Great Aunt's century-long life, she had never been robbed. The volume of jewelry—some worth a quarter at a yard sale and some worth considerably more—was completely overwhelming. Charlotte took a black Sharpie marker and made a sticky note for each of Clara's seven nieces, and the sorting began. Hour after hour, Charlotte held up jewelry—like a gold necklace. I consulted Clara's list and looked up "gold necklace with cross." Char would then move it to Aunt Sarah's growing pile. To finish this job in anything close to an hour, Aunt Clara would have needed to leave us the Harry Potter wand, or at least the Sorting Hat. No such luck.

Aunt Helen's daughter, Barbara, had retired to Florida and was to receive a butterfly broche. A beaded necklace for Marcus's daughter, Marceita, also retired to Florida. Over the course of the summer, Charlotte wrapped some two hundred pieces of jewelry in tissue paper and put them in the correct niece's Ziplock bag. Charlotte had her ears pierced that summer, and I watched her admiring a pair of art deco sapphire earrings. I wished that Aunt Clara's great-great niece Charlotte could have made the list just one time.

Thankfully, Aunt Clara's will stated to sell everything else. Enough time had been spent wrapping bling in tissue paper. We began meeting with estate sale people. I had no concept that "Yard Sale" had become its own industry. We settled on Mr. Johnson with Fini, appropriately named for a company specializing in final Yard Sales finishing off a life's accumulation. Mr. Johnson's agreement was to keep a percentage of the sale and, much more importantly, to take whatever didn't sell to auction, leaving the house's empty rooms broom-clean. A large man with encyclopedic knowledge of stuff, Mr. Johnson should have been a celebrity on Antique Road Show. His crew spent considerable time going through cabinets and drawers, displaying each book and tea towel as if museum-quality, pricing them "to our advantage."

I thought a yard sale would be easy—slap a price tag on everything and sell it Dollar Store style. But the operation was much, much more complex. Who knew that Aunt Clara's Kentucky Derby highball glasses that sat on the bar next to the bourbon were from the legendary race where Secretariat won the Triple Crown? Who knew that my spinster aunt apparently drove to the Derby with Aunt Kate, placed her bet on Secretariat and won? Sure I knew she could play "Camp Town Races" on the ukulele, but little did I know that St. Clara once bet and won at the track. No wonder she needed such a large supply of jewelry, scarves and hats. Mr. Johnson advised it was a good bet the Derby glasses were worth more than a dollar. In the cupboard sat a box of magazines next to a stack of blue china plates that had been purchased with Green Stamps, the original customer loyalty and rewards program. Who knew the box held perfectly preserved *LIFE* magazines with celebs like JFK on their covers? And so it goes with stuff.

Through this Yard Sale process, I realized that housekeeping is really stuff keeping. And Mr. Johnson had his hands full. He sold and dispersed all stuff—clothing, furniture, books—and recorded every sale in line item detail for the estate lawyers. When I came to the house for the last time to meet him, the only thing left was money plant—dried translucent flowers, shiny like silver coins from my great grandmother's yard. Blown from the trash pile, I picked up the ancient bundle. The family money plant always lived in a blue vase by the fireplace. I remember because I once broke the handle on that vase, a mistake of large proportion.

When the Yard Sale concluded and all the trash had been taken out, my family's money was all that remained to fight about ... like spoils of a Civil War.

It was no surprise that Clara left money to charity to help others. She left money to schools in the mountains of Kentucky, and the checks were to be delivered in person. Ouch. Time was my most precious commodity, and driving to the mountains of Kentucky was not exactly on my agenda. My good friend, Doug, is from a nearby town in West Virginia on the Kentucky border with the dubious distinction of being home to the Hatfields and McCoys. I thought he might be interested in a road trip back home to see Mountain Mama, West Virginia. I asked if he was up for it; it took exactly one second to get the "No."

I looked at my work schedule and saw that in October I would be attending a meeting at our office in Roanoke, Virginia. From Roanoke heading west on 64, I could drive across the mountains and get to Hindman, Kentucky, in four to five hours. That was the best I could do. Of course playing Santa and handing out checks for kids in need was not a bad day's work, but it would require me to miss a day of work and take "vacation." I had never been to Hindman, but had heard stories about my mother and her siblings and cousins spending summers there and nearly dying of boredom staying with Big Grandmother and Little Grandmother. After all, they had moved to Lexington and become city kids.

I kept driving my Highlander west from Roanoke toward Wise County, Virginia, listening to Robert Plant, Bob Dylan, Jerry Garcia. I recalled a quote of Jerry's that seemed to summarize all the "tending to" I was now doing: "Somebody has to do something. It's just incredibly pathetic that it has to be us." I laughed out loud. On this strange trip, I turned north on highway 23 and headed into Thomas Jefferson National Forest. In the light all shining on me, the ancient Appalachian Mountains appeared blue. I wound through the mountains and turned onto 119 near Daniel Boone National Forest on the way to Hindman, where my aunt had been born a century ago. Lying in bed the last week of her long life, her nurse remarked that she was still as strong as five women. Her niece, Charlotte, was no different.

As I pulled into Hindman for the first time, I knew it immediately. I crossed the bridge and saw Napier Pharmacy owned by a random cousin, pulled over and parked on the right side of the road. The town was exactly as Aunt Clara described. I saw the Baptist Church and the road leading up the hill behind it. There was no sign, but I knew the road leading to the place where my great grandparents—Caloway and Sarah—ran a hotel and were buried. As if I had been coming to Hindman all my life, I walked up the hill and, as expected, the cemetery was on the right. Without a single misstep on this strange journey, the first gravestone I saw through the fence was etched with the names Caloway and Sarah Napier. I paused and studied other gravestones, including a son who died as an infant, Aunt Clara's brother. Caloway's children, grandchildren and great-grandchildren were a well-educated lot: educators and professors, scientists, doctors, lawyers. I turned and saw where the hotel used to stand and headed down the hill for lunch.

Today Hindman is a small mountain town with art galleries, craft shops and restaurants. Entering a café/gallery, I ordered a country ham sandwich and sat in a cane chair overlooking Troublesome Creek. How many stories had I heard about the dangers of flash flooding at Troublesome Creek? As I ate by the peaceful sounds of the mountain stream, I thought about Great-Grandmother Sarah with genius flowing in her blood. She contributed to the gene pool that contained the very genes that made my mother brilliant, made her beautiful, made her grow tall, made her alive. It also contained the troublesome genes that eventually turned on my mother, slowly diminishing her, destroying one brain cell after another.

After lunch, I crossed the street and headed to the Hindman Settlement School to give away money. I had called the school a couple of weeks in advance, but the person in charge of fundraising was going to be out of town. Since it was the only afternoon I could make work, I met with an administrator instead, who gave me a tour. She asked, "And to whom are you related?" It was a fair question, and I explained that Clara Napier was my great aunt. The administrator asked more questions about my family tree. "Now who, exactly, were Clara's grandparents and great-grandparents?" I explained that I was not the historian in the family. But I thought her great-grandfather was named after an Old Testament prophet or king like Solomon or Moses or something like that. Fitting since Aunt Clara served as our matriarchal saint figure. The administrator stopped dead in her tracks.

"Solomon Everidge? Uncle Sol?"

"Yes. That's right." She hugged me; I wished the check was bigger.

She put her arm in mine and said, "Uncle Sol is our founding father. The Settlement School is a National Historic Site." She went on to relay that the school my great-great-great-grandfather had founded on the side of a mountain was the single most successful pioneer log cabin Settlement School in the Appalachian Mountains and served as the educational model for the public school system in Kentucky and the South. "There is genius coupled with drive in your family. You have some very successful relatives."

She took me to the log cabin on the National Registry of Historic Places, Uncle Sol's home. Perfectly preserved, the log cabin contained original beds covered in quilts, a spinning wheel, fireplace and kitchen table with cane chairs. She showed me an oil painting of Solomon Everidge, at which point I became one hundred percent certain he was indeed my ancestor. His facial features and eyes were the same as Clara's. She showed me a photograph of an oil painting, another familiar face. "I believe her name is Catty. Great Aunt Vena painted the original picture, and it used to hang in my mother's house." Another hug.

In the hills of Eastern Kentucky, Uncle Sol served as the change agent. In his eighties, he walked barefoot more than twenty miles over the mountain to meet two teachers he had heard about who had come for a summer to help educate mountain kids. These two women defined themselves as "reformers"—Katherine Pettit and May Stone from Wellesley College near Boston, Massachusetts. They were part of the Progressive Movement and believed that education was "the lever of social change and at the center of the struggle for a better life."[*]

In time, Uncle Sol recruited these two teachers to begin a school near the fork of Troublesome Creek, so that the mountain kids could be educated. This Settlement School was where my mother's family was educated before they each left Hindman for colleges and universities, including Wellesley, Harvard, Tufts, and University of Kentucky. My mother's kinfolk were straight-A students.

Miss Mary's parents, Robert and Jewel Compton, met while they were both students at The Hindman Settlement School, and the high school sweethearts eventually married. They lived in Hindman with little hope for a future in the small mountain town with little economy. A college

---

[*] Jess Stoddart. *Challenge and Change in Appalachia: The Story of Hindman Settlement School.* Lexington, Kentucky: University Press of Kentucky, 2002, 15.

professor came to Hindman to visit my grandfather as a young man and encouraged him to attend the University of Kentucky. Top graduates of the Hindman Settlement School—like Robert and Jewel—would be admitted to UK and likely receive a scholarship. My grandfather listened. He decided to make the change.

In 1928, Robert loaded his truck with a big dream. On board were his young son Bobby, his wife—pregnant with my mother, some furniture and bedding, trunks of clothes and dishes. Jewel packed salt-cured country hams, smoked turkey, coffee, Ball jars with canned beans, tomatoes and apples. The young family headed 150 miles west to the college town of Lexington with the hope of education and a better life. When my mother, Mary Compton McMullin, died at age eighty-four, she had fulfilled this dream in full in one generation. No time for dilly dally.

This classic image—a rusted truck carrying a young family's dreams, winding down a mountain dirt road headed for the college town—captures the essence of my mother. Still safe inside her mother's womb, this trip was a defining moment in her life. From early on, Miss Mary was moving forward. She was born doing the right thing. She was born unafraid of challenge and expectation. She was born with education, family and faith as driving forces. She would later say, "You make your life." Miss Mary made and lived a remarkable life.

Not long after moving, my mother was born at home on a frigid January 22 in 1929. And about a year later, her sister, Peggy, was born, prematurely, the tiny being so small she fit in her mother's hand. The doctor advised to not get attached to this one. My grandmother ignored this advice and instead visualized Peggy growing and thriving into adulthood. With determination, Jewel fed Peggy around the clock by dipping the edge of a handkerchief in milk and letting the beads of milk drop into her mouth. The baby lived and eventually as a young woman grew to be five foot ten, the tallest of all the Compton women.

A few years later, Sarah was born. Then Linda. Mary was one of five children, the oldest of four daughters. Each one of the look-a-like Compton girls was as striking as the next: tall, with thick black hair, brown eyes, high cheekbones, flawless skin and an inborn sense of fashion. As descendants of Uncle Sol and the Settlement School, these were women who graduated at the top of their high school classes, became Wildcats at the University of Kentucky and pursued advanced degrees—math, education, law and of course, fashion design. Miss Mary is the only person I know who triple majored in college and was awarded a special degree with honors. She and her sisters were expected to use their gifts, to work hard and excel. I asked her once if it was hard growing up with such high expectations. With no hesitation, she responded, "Expect nothing. Get nothing." As an adult, Mary became a champion golf and bridge player. She would beat the women and then beat the men. And for good measure, she would beat them again, without apology. She was born with the spirit of a champion.

We laughed hard at the stories of my mom and her sisters growing up together. Peggy referred to my mom as "Queen Mary," and once told me, "Mary was so smart and so pretty, she could do no wrong in Mother's eyes. In high school, Sarah would wash the sweater and skirt, I would iron them, and Mary would wear them. And then stretch out the sweater!"

Once in elementary school, Mary was chosen to represent the school for a special award. On the day of the event, Mary stood next to her teacher to receive the award. Underneath her new dress, specially made by her mother for the occasion, she wore something called "bloomers" over her underwear.

That morning getting dressed in a hurry, she mistook one of her sister's bloomers for her own. As she stood there with her hand outstretched for the award, the wrong bloomers slid down her legs to her patent leather shoes. Small wonder I grew up to drop trou with the best of them.

As girls, Mary and Peggy shared a room and a double bed. At night, they could hear the radio in the living room, and sometimes, they could hear the radio sign off for the night. As the National Anthem closed the broadcast, Peggy would stand up in the bed, wrap the quilts around her and salute the flag. In the moment of patriotism, Queen Mary was left lying in the bed freezing, kicking and squawking.

12
Bat-Shit Crazy

In Mom's last stages of Alzheimer's, I was never exactly sure what I'd find when I went to visit. Often I was met with a scramble of thought, emotion or movement: standing then sitting, up then down, over and over again. Sometimes she would be in a faraway place unavailable to me. Other times she seemed to be coming undone and anxiety ruled the day. If I showed her a photograph on my iPhone of James and Charlotte and told the picture's story, she would likely engage and return to us for a while. On some weekdays, I would come during my lunch break and help her to focus on eating her meal. And other times she needed no assistance at all and was right there with me.

Both of my parents went to the basketball powerhouse University of Kentucky, my mom on scholarship and my dad on President Roosevelt's G.I. Bill. In 2012 when the Wildcats were in the Final 4 of the NCAA, I watched it on TV with Miss Mary as UK took on Louisville. The old routine of watching UK play basketball brought her home to her true self. As we watched the game, she remembered basketball vividly, recalling the refs' signs for fouls and speaking about defensive strategy. She ordered a Coke from the nurse, as if we were sitting in the stands. We watched and cheered.

She recounted the story of when she was nineteen, and UK played University of Louisville in another basketball final in 1948. Mary asked her mother if she could go to Louisville to watch the game and spend the night. Surprisingly, Jewel had said yes. With her sorority sisters, they loaded into cars and headed to the game to cheer UK to victory. After the game, they spent the night in a hotel before driving home to Lexington in the morning. "My mother never gave me a curfew. The other girls had one. I asked Mother why I didn't have a set time to be home," reflected Miss Mary. "You know when it is time to come home," responded Jewel.

Miss Mary continued, "I never broke my mother's trust. She raised me to do the right thing... despite the mixed results. I loved her and respected her. You know she died of Alzheimer's. Bedridden for years. Doctors are paid to fix you, but they can't fix that one. You can't beat Alzheimer's. You do the right thing and play the best you can, knowing Alzheimer's will care not and beat you in the end."

The nurse returned, "Miss Mary, you have such beautiful children and grandchildren. They are so nice and get along so well." Miss Mary turned her head and laughed, "Boy, do they have you fooled! Kentucky plays like a team. But not MY children." Madness at its finest.

My mother was right. UK did play as a team. But my brother, sister and I were not even on the same playing field. To play on a team like Kentucky, the players leave their individual egos at the gym door. That wasn't possible with us. Too many agendas. Too many dynamics. Too much disrespect to play well with others. Babe Ruth summed up the classic dysfunctional team when he said that "the way a team plays as a whole determines its success. You may have the greatest bunch of individual stars in the world, but if they don't play together, the club won't be worth a dime."

As a teenager when my older brother went away to college, he left home for good. He had no plans to return to Smallville, Virginia. He became a successful finance executive in Atlanta, and most years he returned home for one full-day visit. Burke was chasing his life dream, and he never pretended to have time for Mary, Bill, or Clara, including no time to attend Clara's funeral.

My sister was the baby of the family and magazine beautiful. She was the all-American cheerleader, homecoming princess, sorority girl. Focusing on pretty, she became a pharmaceutical sales rep for Botox until retiring in her early forties to the West End of Richmond, a comfortable environment for Country Club Republicans and evangelical Christians.

My mother and father knew that their children were as different as chalk and cheese. To her credit, Miss Mary kept us together by force of will. A core value for women of her generation was the hold-the-family-together ethic. During the Depression, a family must stick together for survival. But Mary's three children required a mother in order to get along. Without her force, there would be no team nor teamwork. Once her house was sold, we would be without a home court. Even if we wanted to try, the team had no place to practice together.

My father knew his kids did not like each other much, and the dynamics concerned him. When I was at the University of Virginia, he sat me down for a talk. He was starting to have health issues including TIA or mini strokes. He said plainly, "Take care of your mother and be fair." Bill didn't waste words. He summarized all of senior care and estate management in eight words. I told him I would. But I was far too young to understand the magnitude and burden of things like "Power of Attorney" and "Medical Directive."

When my father was growing up in Lexington, his Uncle Don owned a farm and trained racehorses. Bill was raised to bet to win. And when he chose not to bet on his oldest son or daughter to take care of his wife, he knew he wasn't playing by the traditional rules of the track. He wagered on an unlikely middle son, knowing that his choice would not make things easy. But in life, he didn't care much about easy. I wish he had.

After my father's death, I thought that if there was an afterlife, and if one day I saw him again, I would be damn sure I was able to look him in the eye and say that I took care of my mother and was fair to the letter and spirit of the law. On the day Miss Mary moved into assisted living at Lakewood Manor, on the way home, I pulled over at the cemetery where he was buried. Standing at his grave, and with tears and snot pouring down my face, I said, "Dad, I did the best I could."

And that is exactly how you take care of a senior with Alzheimer's. You stumble through and do the best you can for today. And when you screw up, you start again the next day and try to do a little better. As a young man in Lexington, Bill once bowled a perfect game with a score of 300. There would be no perfect game or perfect score with caregiving for Alzheimer's dementia. The best I could do— the best anyone can do—is to keep at it and try to keep the ball out of the gutter for today.

* * *

Before Martha Poppins disappeared from our lives, her parting advice was that Miss Mary would likely need her lawyer, Paul Izzo, to manage her affairs. When the day came to meet about Miss Mary's estate and the sale of her house, she called a cab herself and was driven from Lakewood Manor to the law firm of ThompsonMcMullan in Shockoe Slip. She rose to the occasion, wore a vibrant green tailored suit and looked the part of a respectable Southern lady. In the pocket of her jacket, she carried a folded letter from her doctor stating that she was not yet wacko. She and her lawyer wanted all children present, and if you couldn't make the time to come downtown, they wanted you on the phone. Miss Mary was feeling trifled with, and it drained her mentally and emotionally.

Burke and Libby chose not to meet face-to-face. Over the phone, my sister made their calculated play. At Burke's prompting, she asked our mother to choose her to be in charge of the finances and to change power of attorney from me to her. Since she doesn't work, she promoted herself as the right person with the time available to work on the finances. Miss Mary did not appreciate being put in the position of choosing between children. It didn't help that this news came over the telephone. The tension her daughter was creating was palpable. Annoyed at the situation, Mary turned to the lawyer and said, "No. Keith will continue, as my husband and I planned." Because I don't get along with my siblings and there is no real communication between us, I had volunteered to step down as power of attorney, several times. But my mother and father repeatedly declined. Now she said, "Keith and I are doing just fine, and we are going to keep on keeping on."

To finalize the sale of her house, Miss Mary's lawyer requested all three children's signatures, as the house was held in trust with the children named as the trustees. My older brother in Atlanta spoke up and began questioning the sale. Miss Mary held the letter from her doctor in her hand. She turned to the lawyer and said, "Dissolve my trust. I'm taking the cash offer for my home." The lawyer said into the phone, "Mrs. McMullin is prepared to dissolve the

McMullin Trust." Burke stammered, "There is no need." If it had been dissolved, I would have been granted total control as acting power of attorney. Burke then requested more costly financial reporting from the law firm and an $11,000 check that, according to his accounting, he had been shorted years earlier from my father's estate. She said wearily, "Give him the money." Her lawyer raised an eyebrow and said that he would check the agreement with Lakewood Manor to ensure that this gift would not break her contract.

After the phone was hung up, the lawyer advised that if I left all of my mother's money exactly where my parents had invested it, my brother and sister would not be able to make a case against me in any court for mismanagement of funds. Paul felt that they would not hesitate to press charges over money and start a Civil War. He had spoken with Miss Mary's financial advisor at Wells Fargo. Barb Dittmeier reported that Wells Fargo leadership would not likely approve of moving or consolidating Miss Mary's money at this time. The tone of Burke's emails had been threatening, and the company could be put at risk of a lawsuit. So Miss Mary's money stayed put, generating a nice low return on investments and short-circuiting greed.

Regardless of my brother and sister's feelings about me, they asked a key question that all families must ask when caring for a senior with dementia. And Miss Mary knew their question: *was she bat-shit crazy?* (Translation: was she mentally competent to make legal and financial decisions for herself?) It wasn't in her nature to give up on life. Ultimately, the decision of competence is made by the attending physician. My mother's doctor, Richard Gergoudis, is regarded as the top geriatric doctor in central Virginia. He explained that "competent" meant my mother should be able "to direct her legal and financial affairs." Not manage them in detail, but direct them. Eventually in 2011, he wrote the letter stating that she was no longer competent, a little more than a year before her death. Until that time, her affairs were directed by her and her alone. In no way did my brother and sister agree, but taking on Dr. Gergoudis in court and arguing sanity's shades of grey would require significant time, energy and money.

When the doctor diagnosed Miss Mary as incompetent, I felt it was amazingly accurate. That summer, I watched my mother as she signed her name for the last time. A signature is a unique expression of who you are, and of course, the tyrant Alzheimer takes that away, too. I was helping Miss Mary write a note to be included with the checks to the beneficiaries of Aunt Clara's estate. She was no longer able to physically hand-write a full-length letter for each person. Looking at her notes, she slowly dictated a letter, and I typed it on my iPad. I read it to her; she concentrated, made edits. Thoughtful and well-mannered until her last day, below are her last written words:

> *Dear Members of Clara's Family,*
>
> *At long last, Clara's estate is finished. It took fourteen months to get her final tax return! In her will, Clara made a generous donation to the Hindman Settlement School and Oneida Institute in Kentucky. It reflected her lifelong love of learning, education and young people. She also gave something to each of you, her nieces and nephews. The check is enclosed.*
>
> *Aunt Clara was such a special person. Even my grandchildren—her great-great nieces and nephew —have fond memories of her singing and playing the ukulele. I always enjoyed living with Clara.*
>
> *Much love,*
> *Mary C. McMullin*

She wanted to sign each love note, but it was unrealistic for her to write her name over and over again. So I printed one letter for her to sign, and we agreed that I would make copies of it to include in the box being mailed to each family member. Miss Mary reached for a Bic pen and practiced signing her name in full. After practicing until she was satisfied with how it looked on the paper, she asked for the letter. With determination, she signed her name one last time. Alzheimer's was gaining ground.

13
Free and Alone

It was a tight squeeze shoehorning so much of life between the ages of forty and fifty. I held some very challenging leadership positions in health care technology, a complex and highly competitive growth industry. I was raising Charlotte and James, which included helping my son with dyslexia to read, write and do school. I got to the leaf raking, to the gym, and to the kids' practices on time—soccer, basketball, swimming, track, lacrosse and field hockey. I provided care to aging senior family members and in time, laid them to rest. I was grateful to be busy with it all alongside my life-partner, Marty, who was surviving her own battle with cancer at the age of forty-three. Small wonder I liked hitting the pause button and drinking a beer at the neighborhood bar or paddling on the James River with DougE.

Some things you carry with you beyond your forties, and other luggage you set down and continue without. At some point, the letting go and leaving behind becomes as defining an act as what you carry forward. Life's journey is far too arduous to play Sherpa. Traveling heavy is deadly.

I remember years ago being at a cocktail party, when one of Miss Mary's girlfriends, enjoying a dirty martini, put her arm in mine and asked, "How is your mother's health?" We talked some about Alzheimer's dementia, the disease that took her mother's life as well. She looked directly at me, and in her deep southern drawl said, "When my mother died, I never felt more free or more alone." I held onto those words, spoken to me from some sort of modern-day prophet wearing pearls of great price. As the people close to me died, I tried to embrace both the freedom and the aloneness experienced with the death of a loved one. Rather than combat aloneness, I let it be.

At Ole Daddy's funeral, my wife's large extended family filled the pews of his Presbyterian church in Atlanta. Hilarious stories about my salty dog of a father-in-law, one after another, made for a memorable service. Uncle Gus, roughly six foot two and 250 pounds, shared a story about Ole Daddy and his love for shooting his sixteen-gauge double-barrel shotgun. To celebrate Christmas day at the farm, he would fill the clay target thrower and shoot skeet off the back porch of the house. The good citizens in the encroaching suburbs weren't too happy about guns being fired in their general direction on Christmas day. Nonetheless, the police weren't interested in arresting Ole Daddy that day or any other day.

Ole Daddy died of Alzheimer's, as did his mother, father and sister. In his final years as he struggled to walk, communicate, eat and remember the people close to him, he remained a crackerjack shot. Even as he suffered with dementia, when he heard the command, "Pull!" he would reach for his shotgun, aim and blow the orange skeet out of the sky. In a millisecond, he could find his balance, shoulder the gun, judge space and time and shoot with precision. We were left dumbfounded. No doctor or scientist would think it possible (or a good idea), but his brain synapses were still able to fire and connect, enabling him to function with the instincts of a pro marksman. Maybe he visualized the clay target as his enemy—Alzheimer's disease itself.

Alzheimer's is the great dis-connector. It distances you from mind, emotions, memory and voice. It separates you from time, space, your personality, and from your friends and family. In Miss Mary's case, the tragedy of Alzheimer's included disconnecting me from my brother and sister. We were like brain cells damaged by Alzheimer's disease. The cells' nerve endings became a tangled mess, broken down, no longer functioning or communicating with one other. We were cells in isolation. The fact that money meant little to Miss Mary and that she had saved a small fortune added fuel to the fire.

The full impact of our failed relationships came to me at Ole Daddy's funeral. As I walked across the cold slate floor of the church after the memorial service, I knew I was alone in my grief. I was only a couple of miles from my brother's house, yet I knew no McMullin would attend, extend a hand or be there for my family. I knew my sibling relationships had extended their shelf life, and if you opened that can, it would only stink. My phone would not ring. No flowers would arrive. No memorial donation would be made. My brother and sister taught me to ask for nothing from them and to expect nothing in return. While leaving the church, I said goodbye not only to Ole Daddy but also to my brother, my sister and my childhood. Alzheimer's doesn't tolerate fairy tale endings.

Eventually I did hear from them. During the week chemo cream covered my head to remove layers of skin with cancer issues, they called my mother's lawyer instructing him to tell me to speed up with the financial reporting, submit additional information they wanted, change her beneficiary documents to "per sterpes" to encompass their children and do this work without compensation. Chop, chop! I laughed hard. If I was to die of skin cancer that night and there were no "per sterpes" clauses, they would have inherited my portion of Miss Mary's savings and could have lived unhappily ever after.

It was a moment of clarity that remains with me today. I knew then that I would not reduce my mother's memory to money. It was surprisingly easy to set down the suitcase full of money, to walk on and not look back. On occasion, I have glanced in the rearview mirror. *If Miss Mary had been penniless and if money and the control of money had not been issues, would her three children have pulled together to care for her?* Who knows? I do know that when Mary's younger sister was lying in a "Medicaid Bed" dying of Alzheimer's and her savings had long been spent on health care, her children were suing one another over the issue of no money. It is not easy to imagine a world where there is no wrestling over money and control.

On the wall by my desk where I managed my mother's finances for years, I taped a picture of my son's red Schwinn Varsity bicycle built for two. James bought it off Craig's List and restored it to its original condition. The $50 he paid for the bike would bring him, Charlotte, and his cousins— my sister's kids—infinitely more happiness riding it in tandem than any battle over $500,000 of my mother's money would ever yield. Miss Mary's four grandkids in Richmond grew up playing together at her home, and they would like each other and be far closer than her own children. It was a remarkable legacy left by a never-give-up champion of love.

14
The Grinch Who Stole Miss Mary

I remember as a kid sitting on khaki-colored carpet at the top of the stairs waiting and waiting for my dad to give the signal. Once we got the thumbs-up and he said in his Southern drawl, "All right now," we would run down the stairs to Christmas morning, jockeying for position. The waiting was hard. I would have been awake for hours in the top bunk, and then at the head of the stairs. I could see Christmas stockings so full of presents they had to be taken from the fireplace and laid in living room chairs. And that was just the beginning. The bounty continued in the adjacent family room, where an abundance of wrapped gifts surrounded our über-decorated Christmas tree. Holy morning in the land of plenty.

The stockings alone provided a full Christmas. One year I opened a Nikon camera, which was nestled inside my red felt stocking, an awesome surprise. My father usually bought some hilarious kitchen gadget off TV, like the ever-popular

Veg-O-Matic. Of course we would then endlessly reenact the commercial, "It slices, it dices, it makes julienne fries. Chop an onion without shedding a tear. Wait, there's more…" And there was more. Mary received the obligatory Mom-gifts: hand cream, dish towels, Opium perfume that came with a Dad wink. It was all wrapped in holiday paper, including some irridiculous present for us kids, like striped gym socks, that no child had ever circled in the Best Products Christmas Catalog.

Even the wrapping of presents was a holiday ritual. I remember my father setting up a card table in front of the television every year in December. Surrounded by a mountain range of bags, boxes, wrapping paper, tags, scissors and tape, he would turn on a Redskins football game for entertainment while wrapping each present. Bill locked the door to the room and then laid out Santa Claus paper, Frosty the Snowman riding-a-sled paper and shiny blue foil paper in a super-sized roll from Reynolds Metals. With an engineer's geometric precision, he expertly cut, folded and taped the corners of each package. It was much later in life when I realized presents could be delivered in a Macy's bag with the receipt right there for an effortless and emotion-free return.

While my father wrapped, my mother spent the season as a good elf in the kitchen. Baking was as fundamental to Our Christmas Story as The Baby Jesus himself. Miss Mary may have been a career gal before her time. She may have had a full-time housekeeper who helped cook during the week. But make no mistake, Julia Child had little on Mary. The smell alone of Christmas cookies baking in the oven was proof. The Three Kings passed out gold, frankincense and myrrh, but please pass me my mom's turtles with home-made caramel, pecan tassies, forgotten foam with little bits of candy cane, oatmeal lace cookies, butter cream mints, divinity and an entire tray of goo bars. Thank you, Jesus.

Born in 1929, Miss Mary grew up long before Betty Crocker had invented boxed cake mix and brownie mix. Grammy Mary began her baking ritual by donning a red Christmas apron and retrieving an ancient grey metal box from the kitchen corner cupboard, jam packed with yellowed recipe cards (long before the days of epicurious.com). She would flip through hundreds of recipes to find, perhaps, *Christmas Sugar Cookies* written in script. The project looked to me like a science experiment spread across every available counter, including the top of the dishwasher, conveniently mounted on caster wheels so that it could be rolled anywhere for additional counter space.

For Miss Mary, cooking was fun. A mess was not an issue. Before the days of microwave ovens, butter was left on the counter to soften to room temperature and then beaten with a hand mixer in a yellow Pyrex bowl. Sugar was sifted and added gradually, the batter beaten until light and fluffy. Room-temperature eggs were cracked over a kitchen bowl and any egg shells were fished out with an old grapefruit spoon, its jagged edges ideal for snagging stray pieces. Eggs were added slowly, properly, one at a time and then vanilla and almond extracts. My job was sifting flour in an ancient cylindrical metal sifter that squeaked when I turned the red wood handle. King Arthur Flour was sifted twice over waxed paper, making perfect white mountains. The flour was added gradually until a stiff dough formed.

Miss Mary separated the dough into balls, her hands flying as she patted the dough flat, spread flour over the kitchen counter in a back-and-forth motion like sowing seeds. She would rub the rolling pin—its handles long missing—with more flour. She would then move the pin back and forth, rolling the dough to an even thickness of one-eighth of an inch. Next we kids used metal cookie cutters, stored in a beat-up wooden canister circa 1800, to cut out shapes: reindeers, angels, Santas, gingerbread boys, Christmas trees, bells and diamonds. Using colored sugar, we decorated each cookie. They were transferred to a crusty metal baking sheet and then popped into the oven. The timer was set. But Grammy Mary relied on her nose. She could tell by smell when cookies were golden brown and ready to come out. We baked dozens of cookies for friends and neighbors and stored them in metal tins in the cool basement. Of course, we always got to pick out our favorites and gobble them up with milk in the Santa mug.

Sugar cookies were only the beginning. Out came double boilers, candy thermometers, cast iron pans and pots of every dimension. One Christmas cookie miracle involved separating and whipping egg whites with a hand beater until a peak formed so high the bowl could no longer contain it. My job was to find all candy canes in the house, unwrap them, dump them in a bag and smash them to smithereens with a hammer on the concrete basement floor. I got to dump the candy cane particles into the egg white goop and fold them in with a red-handled spatula. The cookies went into the oven for the entire night and in the morning, yum. One year someone at the office gave my father the mother lode of all candy canes, probably two feet tall and two inches in diameter. I was instructed to bash it to bits, and we made candy cane ice cream with the hand-crank ice cream maker. And out of a double-boiler apparatus on the back burner of the stove came hot fudge to drizzle on top.

To me, Christmas was about scarfing an abundance of cookies. To my parents and Great Aunt Clara, it centered more around The Baby Jesus, as recounted in Luke. Not Matthew, Mark or John. My mother was thirty-six and my father thirty-seven when I was born in 1965. They were ten years older than my friends' parents and belonged to the Greatest Generation with little awareness of the Me

Generation. All in all, my parents did "the right thing," including going to church most Sundays. At Christmas, Advent wreaths, Advent calendars, crèches, Handel's Messiah and the sacred Christmas Eve service stood as givens.

One year, it was my job to take Great Aunt Clara to the Christmas Eve service. Not a day less than eighty-five and still good-looking, Aunt Clara had her hair and nails done for the occasion. She wore an emerald green dress with a scarf resembling stained glass and adorned with a holly wreath pin. In the car with the heat on high and windows closed tight, a smell far greater than its parts of perfume, hairspray and powder lingered in the air. We arrived early to ensure a good seat. Aunt Clara liked to go to the family service, the one where kids act out a white suburban version of the Christmas story. Not to be confused with the literal Bible story of a mid-Eastern family in crisis, the one with Mary, an unwed Jewish teenager about fourteen years old, nine months pregnant and broke, catching a ride on an ass for a quick trip away from her home with her much-older embarrassed boyfriend.

The preferred version focused on cute white kids dressed as adorable sheep, cows, and blond angels wearing crooked halos made of pipe cleaners and glitter. Aunt Clara and I found seats in the wooden church pew, and we stood and sang hymns with sweet visions of "The Little Lord Jesus Asleep in the Hay." Mary, dressed in a plush bathrobe, and Joseph, wearing a poncho and holding a large cane, walked down the aisle behind a snickering ten year old in an Eeyore the Donkey costume left over from Halloween. They eventually made it to the front of the church with paparazzi grandparents in close pursuit. Joseph walked up the two steps in the front of the sanctuary and knocked mime-style on the imaginary door of The Bethlehem Inn.

The Inn Keeper, in striped bathrobe and do-rag, opened the imaginary door. Joseph offered a smooth lie, "Do you

have a room for my wife and me? She is heavy with child."
To which the Inn Keeper responded, "There's no room at
the Inn... but won't you come in for a drink?" Aunt Clara
laughed until she cried. Toward the end of the service, it was
time to sing the favorite hymn "Silent Night." When the
refrain began, "Silent night, holy night, sleep in heavenly
peace," everyone raised a mini flashlight in the shape of a
candle. We lifted the glow sticks like shot glasses to celebrate
the birth of The Baby Jesus. At the song's conclusion, we
turned to those next to us for the offering of peace. Devout
and respectable Aunt Clara, wielding her mini light saber in
one hand, extended her other hand to her neighbor, looked
him directly in the eye and deadpanned, "May the force be
with you."

After the service, we headed home for a drink and
Christmas Eve dinner. As was her tradition, Miss Mary
had been focusing on her food ministry. Having cooked for
days, family and friends now gathered around Miss Mary's
dining room table to enjoy her legendary meal. With everyone seated, Miss Mary, in red apron and lipstick, opened
the door of The Magic Oven and about a hundred hot and
delicious dishes commenced to the table. Like a scene out
of Harry Potter, the food magically kept coming: sweet
potato casserole, green beans almondine, Party Potatoes,
corn pudding, stuffing, turkey and country ham. Just when
I thought the table and sideboard could hold no more food,
Miss Mary jumped up and said, "Good heavens! Where are
the oysters?" Next thing you knew, a piping hot pan of delicious oysters hit the table. And then ambrosia, a crazy good
fruit concoction, emerged, leaving just enough room for hot
buttered White House rolls and cranberry relish. Let the
red wine pour.

Miss Mary's white coconut cake with a holly sprig on top
was displayed in plain view so that everyone knew what was

yet to come. While the coffee percolated in preparation for dessert, Miss Mary asked, "Now who would like seconds?" It was easy to show your love for her—just eat a second helping.

As she grew older, Miss Mary's grandkids became the focus of her holidays. She liked to slip to the kids' table, where she explained that she had made the sweet potatoes with marshmallows, so it was really a form of early dessert. All the picky eaters gobbled up another helping. After dinner, she would lean over to her oldest grandchild, "Charlotte, please bring me a present. Hurry!" Long-legged Charlotte sprinted to the tree.

When Charlotte was about four years old, she wore black velvet pants and a red silk coat from Aunt Bunny in Hong Kong for Christmas Eve dinner. Charlotte picked a matching outfit for Grammy Mary to wear, black pants and an absurd red Christmas sweater with sparkle trees and jingle bells. In the family room with the Christmas tree, Charlotte pushed "play" on Miss Mary's CD player and out blasted California Christmas with The Beach Boys singing about Rudolph.

There was nothing Miss Mary loved more than an invitation to dance. Charlotte and Grammy jitterbugged the night away with Charlotte's blonde hair swinging and my mother's head thrown back laughing out loud, fully engaged in the moment.

This is the Miss Mary that the intruder Alzheimer's broke into our lives to steal. But try as it might, Alzheimer's could no more take the spirit of Miss Mary than The Grinch could steal the spirit of Christmas. When asked if she believed in Santa, my mother dependably answered, "I feel sorry for people who only believe in things they can see. Can you see God? Can you see love? I believe in the spirit of Christmas." She taught us to believe from the heart.

* * *

During the last year of my mother's life, the kids and I drove to Lakewood manor a few weeks before Christmas. James and Grammy Mary wanted to go for a drive to see Richmond's Tacky Light Tour and houses covered in millions of Christmas lights, apparently visible from space. My own home was now included—James had illuminated it for the universe.

We parked and the kids ran down the sidewalk to see Grammy, the glass doors sliding open and the water sculpture gurgling. They ran down her hall, turning left at the painting of red poppies, and entered her quiet room, taking over the stillness with loud voices, excitement and hugs. Charlotte and James helped her stand and put on her long winter coat and matching black leather gloves. We transferred her to the wheel chair, helping her step backward until the back of her legs touched the edge of the seat and then lowered her to a sitting position. Charlotte, growing tall as a supermodel with a thick mane of hair, kneeled and moved each of Grammy's feet onto a chair pedal. Charlotte and James talked nonstop about school friends, basketball games and Christmas lights. Grammy listened intently and gazed at them from a faraway place, smiling and trying to keep up with their words. James signed her out at the nurse's station, and we pushed her chair to the car to transfer her again. Grammy was confused about next steps, but with help, sat in the front passenger seat. Charlotte helped move her feet, clad in sensible SAS black leather shoes, inside the car. I cranked the heat until James squawked that his tennis shoes were melting.

Words came slowly to Grammy Mary, but she found the words to ask James about the light tour. We drove past Westhampton Memorial Park, and James and Charlotte waved and exclaimed, "Hello, Poppy!" Just over Jesus' left shoulder was where we had buried my father ten years earlier with the government-issued grave marker for World War II vets. My mother used to joke that it was her very favorite plastic flower farm. We turned left on Maybeury and looked at a house covered in multicolored lights reflecting off the lake. Miss Mary stared forward, her movements stiff; that night she was unable to rotate her head. We passed another house covered from roof to yard with dancing lights, inflatable snowmen and Santas. The Grinch. Miss Mary only smiled and said, "It's time for me to go home now. Thank you."

"Of course," I said, silencing grumbles about a dozen more houses to see. That was all the Christmas she could manage.

A few days later, we loaded up the car with our kids and their cousins to have dinner with Grammy Mary at Lakewood's dining room. We ordered off the menu and the bill was added to Mother's monthly tab. She was still providing for us. Grandkids sitting around the table talked a mile a minute, cutting up and laughing. Each showed iPhone pictures to Grammy, telling the image's story.

Miss Mary sat in her black wheelchair at the head of the table. She struggled for words and nodded occasionally. I ordered for us both: steamship round, sweet potatoes and broccoli. James would help cut her meat, and with queuing, she could still feed herself. There was some general confusion about when to use a fork and when to use a a spoon. Her hand quivered as she guided the straw to her lips for sips of iced tea.

The waiters arrived with everyone's order. Grammy Mary extended her hands to James and Charlotte. We all held hands. The ancient Scottish Warrior bowed her head and from a sacred drawer pulled out a prayer, "Lord, thank you for this which we are about to receive and for our many blessings."

To celebrate Christmas and her final year in the final stages of Alzheimer's, Miss Mary led us all in heartfelt gratitude. Stop the insanity.

* * *

How does one singlehandedly cook a feast for a dozen people the night before Christmas? Miss Mary's brain was able to plan the recipes, purchase the ingredients at Ukrop's Super Market, anticipate the sequential steps, juggle the preparation and serve ten dishes piping hot from The Magic Oven at 7:00 p.m. on the dot.

What happens inside Miss Mary's brain for her to successfully cook a feast? Picture her standing in the center of her kitchen. She is wearing her red Christmas apron and is in full action, surrounded by cabinets and drawers and appliances. She knows instinctively what to do: flour from the corner cupboard, slotted spoon in the top drawer on the right, cream on the refrigerator door.

A healthy brain operates in similar fashion. In a sense, the brain houses thousands of cabinets, cupboards, drawers. The hippocampus, the central conductor in the brain, functions like Miss Mary, pulling information from various storage areas, combining data and acting in a flash. To make a batch of Christmas cookies, the central conductor of the brain extracts what it needs from the right storage area. From one drawer she pulls the memorized list of ingredients, like flour, sugar and butter. From another drawer the recall of sequential steps, like adding eggs, one at a time. From another cabinet, the memory of how the dough should feel when it is ready to be rolled out.

The neurons within the brain communicate with one another and relay information throughout the body. The synapses, or communication points between brain cells, work together in perfect synchronization. Neurotransmitters, such as acetylcholine, guide the functions of attention and memory. The transmitter dopamine connects thoughts to physical movement, telling the hands to open the oven door and remove the cookie sheet. The brain is the most intricate and mysterious organ in the body. However complex the workings of the brain, it is dependent on the nerve synapses of each brain cell communicating with one another and relaying information throughout the body. This rapid-fire communication system is what enables a human to bake Christmas cookies.

Alzheimer's disease targets and destroys these nerve synapses, generating havoc within the brain. One by one, each brain cell's synapses become tangled and discombobulated. The communication point is lost. Alzheimer's is a communication breakdown. The brain cells are isolated from one another, then whither and die. As more and more brain cells fail to communicate and function, the patient loses her ability to communicate and function. Like an individual brain cell, she is isolated and no longer connected to other people. The high performer becomes the slow responder. Eventually, after a couple billion nerve cells die, the brain no longer effectively tells the throat to swallow. Alzheimer's dementia comes with a performance guarantee: confusion, isolation, slow death.

15
The Waiting Room

I remember being about four years old, waking up early before the sunrise and hearing my dad begin the morning coffee-making ritual. He lifted off the lid of the stainless steel percolator with black handle, scooped Eight O'Clock Coffee out of the aluminum canister, loaded the cylindrical metal filter, turned on the kitchen water faucet to fill the pot and plugged it in. The kitchen clock made a mechanical sound as it struck 6:00 a.m. Something about the gurgle of the coffee as it swirled inside the glass knob on top of that percolator would nudge me out of bed.

I would sneak down the stairs to the kitchen just to see the coffee pot's small red light. In 1969, this was the only appliance light in the house. Recently, I got up at 4:30 a.m. to let out Abner, the barking beagle. While stumbling around in my boxers, I counted thirty seven flashing lights before I got the barking beagle the hell out of the house: clocks, iPhones, TVs, WiFi, aquarium, charger, microwave oven and yes, the coffee pot. In 1969, not only were there no digital lights, there was no high-def flat screen smart TV. In the Dark Ages before the dawn of Digital Light, I would follow my dad downstairs to our TV, which resided in an enormous box with faux wood paneling, its own piece of furniture. The black and white TV image included snow zigzagging across the screen and an enormous rabbit ear antenna on top, in perpetual need of adjustment.

My father, the World War II Navy man, rose early for his daily exercises in grey sweat pants and a white t-shirt: push-ups, sit ups, military presses, rounds of jumping rope. A man of his time, he golfed, bowled and played bridge, winning titles in each.

My dad liked to turn on "Sailor Bob" on channel WRVA (W Richmond VA) for me to watch from the sofa while he worked out. This homegrown TV show featured Sailor Bob in a white Navy uniform and sailor hat. While Bob told a story, he drew it with a black magic marker. Before Sesame Street and Oscar the Grouch came on the scene, my TV friends were artist Sailor Bob and his kooky puppets, like zany Gilly Gull and madcap Sparky, who were always good for an early morning knock-knock joke.

The show's highlight was a black-and-white reel of "Popeye the Sailor Man." This spinach eating, bicep bulging, corncob pipe-smoking cartoon character was in the business of saving his slightly anorexic girlfriend, Olive Oyl, on a daily basis. Although I had not yet met an anorexic woman named after a food and who seemed in constant peril, Popeye became our tattooed hero anyway. After the cartoon ended, I would climb on top of my pop's back for his Popeye Challenge. And he would knock out another set of push-ups while I laughed loudly, the extra weight no issue for him.

Some thirty years later when my son was about three years old, my parents and I agreed that I would come over early, at 7:00 a.m., on a Saturday to help with finances. Rather than wake up and make the coffee like my dad, I drove by Starbucks, or Fivebucks as my father referred to it. Drinking my Grande Sumatra Bold, I pulled the Volvo station wagon into the driveway and walked to the front door. When I rang the doorbell, Miss Mary opened the door in a frantic rush. She had already been to Ukrop's Super Market to buy the day-old items on super sale. When she returned home, something was not right with my father. He wasn't well. She was dialing 911.

I headed down the stairs to the family room, the same stairs I had run down to watch all those episodes of "Sailor Bob" and "Popeye." My father slept in a hospital bed now and required care for Parkinson's and the effects of multiple strokes. The drapes were drawn closed. I walked to his bed and put my hand on his shoulder. "Dad, it's me, Keith." But his body was stiff. I put my hand on his forehead; it was cold as stone. His lips were blue. My father was dead.

I turned and went back up the stairs. In as steady a voice I could summon, I said, "Mama, Dad is dead." Hugging her, an ocean of emotion swirled and tears and snot poured forth. My father, her life partner of more than fifty years, had died during his sleep, just as his mother had.

We were both crying and in shock when the ambulance pulled into the driveway, its diesel engine rumbling. Suddenly, medics surrounded us. Great Aunt Clara came down the stairs in her robe, and my mother delivered the news. "Clara, Bill has died." Aunt Clara cried out with a mourner's wail, and two of the most independent and strong-willed women I knew, hugged and sobbed. In the middle of unrelenting waves of emotion, the medics needed us to answer questions. They were required to ask about medications, illness and potential foul play. We responded, and my father's death was documented in black ink. They explained they would not be taking "the body" as there was nothing a doctor could do for it at the hospital.

The funeral home, about a mile from my mom and dad's house, had been notified. Within minutes a long black hearse backed up the driveway. It was not yet 7:30 in the morning, and a hearse had come for my father's dead body. I moved past the crowd of noisy strangers in the family room, the medics and drivers. I bent down to my father and said, "I love you, Daddy. Goodbye." I kissed his forehead, his skin cold to the touch of my lips, his life energy no longer there.

* * *

Several years later, I stood in my mother's kitchen, and I heard singing and dancing in the same downstairs family room. I opened the door and headed down. Great Aunt Clara, age ninety-nine, was sitting in the green velveteen Med-Lift reclining chair. Ukulele in hand, Clara played songs-by-request for her great-great-nieces and nephews. Charlotte, James, Emily, and Caroline danced around the family room as Clara sang, "Five foot two, eyes are blue. Oh what those five feet can do! Has anybody seen my gal?" More hit songs by request followed with more dancing. More laughing.

The next day, I returned to see Mom and Clara. With the hospice nurse in the room, Clara asked me "Is it time to cross the river?" She was fading. For the first time in ninety-nine years, she needed to be carried to bed. I picked her up and settled her, noticing the years had not diminished her beauty. I ignored the mystery of her question and answered simply, "Yes."

But what, exactly, was Clara asking? Was she asking King David's eternal question, "When will I see God's face?" Was she asking if it was time to cross the River Jordan to see Jesus coming with arms outstretched?

Or was she asking if it was time to cross the James River and head to Dillard's Department Store at Stony Point Mall? Was she thinking about dress shopping one last time to look her very best as she crossed the threshold of death's door into the unknown?

I have no idea. God or Fashion? It was a toss-up.

Aunt Clara's death was peaceful, spiritual, a holy place. The presence of angels was tangible. She would have described the experience as being a "thin place," the narrow space dividing this world and the spiritual. Like looking through the shears that hung in her room's window: you see a blurred image distinct enough to offer a sense of what's there. Profoundly at peace, Aunt Clara was in bed five days before she died. She would often reach out her arms, lean upward toward heaven and say the names of long dead relatives. She lived in this state, in the angels' waiting room, those five days. I halfway expected her to ascend in a whirl of white hospital sheets with the ceiling opening wide to vibrant blue sky above, white ceiling tiles and puffy clouds swirling and Jesus himself swinging low for Saint Clara aboard his sweet chariot, ablaze like the sun.

On the last day, her lungs began to fill with fluid. Her mouth opened slightly, and a gurgling sound replaced her breath. The hospice nurse called me early on a Friday morning as I drove to work. I turned around and went straight to the house. Miss Mary and I shared with Clara that we loved her, and Charlotte and James would tell the story of her remarkable life for another hundred years. In the morning light, she breathed her last, and the spirit passed through every cell like a breeze. Her father, Caloway, was born before the Civil War. My kids' immediate family history had always stretched to the Civil War. With our Greatest Aunt's death came the end of an era—The Clara Era—of which we were privileged to play a part.

My father died unexpectedly during his sleep. My great Aunt Clara's body wore out after ninety-nine years of use. Death by Alzheimer's is different. The disease shows no mercy and would never permit an unexpected quick death or a respectable passing from old age. Alzheimer's, the merciless tyrant, demands a slow and tortured death sentence. Its victims sit on death row waiting for years, as one brain cell after another fades and dies. The human brain has billions of nerve cells, more than the night sky has stars. One by one, the stars go dark, their light and energy extinguished. Darkness and death descend like a pitch-black sky without star or moon.

For my mom, death came over many years. We counted down the seven stages of Alzheimer's dementia, like counting strokes when paddling a kayak shell, one stroke after the next. We kept counting and moving toward the shore on this unplanned trip to the end. When Miss Mary entered the seventh stage of the disease, she required full care at Lakewood Manor. The truth of the matter is you want to stop counting, you don't wish another day of Alzheimer's on a fellow human being. You find yourself hoping for death, wishing for death, praying for death as an act of mercy for your brilliant and kindhearted mother.

Eventually, the wait ends. I was in a meeting when Gladys called. "Lakewood Nurse Station" appeared on my iPhone. The nurse's words stopped me cold: "Miss Mary is nonresponsive." I flashed back to the image of my mother kicking off her shoes and dancing barefoot with Charlotte, head thrown back, laughing out loud, fully engaged in life. A supernova was flickering.

Miss Mary would not be "responsive" again. She lay in the hospital bed with white sheets and blankets covering her slim body, eyes closed, breath slow. Her smooth skin and silver hair shone beautifully in early morning light. It was time to say goodbye. Her medical directive on file with Lakewood

Manor was written plainly: Miss Mary wanted her right to death. She did not want to be kept alive by machines or tubes or something called "thickened water." Quiet and peaceful, she moved toward death. When the wait wasn't so easy, the hospice nurse eased Mom's pain with morphine.

Miss Mary had outlived most of her family and friends. She had seen death up close many times and was comfortable with it. My good friend and kayak buddy, Dr. Dave, is a neurologist and brain injury expert. He offered to read my mother's MRI tests and give a second opinion, a true kindness. He confirmed that her Alzheimer's was in the final stage. The MRI revealed multiple strokes and severe damage at the base of what remained of her brain. This brain stem area controls basic body functions like breathing. Miss Mary would die in a matter of days. Dr. Dave offered to answer any questions family members might want to ask him. No questions remained.

A simple truth about the last week of life: each day holds twenty-four hours, and friends and family generally want to visit between 9:00 a.m. and 5:00 p.m. This is only an eight-hour window of time, leaving sixteen hours each day for me to be alone with Miss Mary, just me and a couple of beeping machines with blinking red lights by her side. The nurses call it the "graveyard shift." It's not nearly as creepy as it sounds.

I brought the kids over as often as they wanted to say goodbye to Grammy Mary. One evening, James asked to see her and hug her one more time. We stood by the bed, but Grammy Mary was restless, stiff-limbed and unable to settle. We put our hands on her arm and tried to soothe her. James told her how special she was and that he would always love her. The hospice nurse entered to help.

Anxious that I had made the wrong decision by bringing James, I apologized when we stepped out of the room, saying I was sorry if he was upset at seeing his grandmother struggle. I asked if it was hard when Grammy didn't seem to hear him or recognize him. James said matter-of-factly, "Grammy's heart has ears." And we drove home like it was any other night, without tears or sniffling, tuning into Jazz in General on the radio. The essential truth about caring for a senior with dementia delivered by a ten-year-old boy who understood. Miss Mary, with the spirit of a champion, had taught her grandchildren that love always wins. We drove home listening to the radio, and Sarah Vaughan sang to us the definition of "always." Forever and a day. Looking out the window, James stated as fact, "Grammy loves me always in her heart—forever and a day."

For me, my mother's last day on earth began at 5:00 a.m. with a smiling African-American nurse's aide asking me, "Baby, what can I get you for breakfast? Coffee? Eggs? Grits? Bacon? Whatever you want." She returned with a Southern-style breakfast, a fitting start to my last day with Mary after countless mornings of bacon and eggs with her. I recalled her green robe, the permanent smell of bacon woven into the fabric.

I ate my generous breakfast, read the newspaper and watched the morning light come shining as my mother slept peacefully. I put my hand on hers and practiced waiting. "I Shall Be Released" by Bob Dylan kept playing through my mind.

The sun rose, and the nurse came by with the coffee pot. It was getting dangerously close to 8:00 a.m., and people would begin coming in and out of the room, busy with their own agendas. I leaned in and said that I was going to head to work for a while and come back later. "Thank you," she uttered. Somehow she found enough voice for a final statement—thank you. Miss Mary remembered her manners.

I worked for a few hours, preparing a launch of a disease-management program, more tools to prevent suffering and save lives. But of course there was nothing I could do to save my mom. No one could beat Alzheimer's. My phone vibrated. The nurse told me it was time. I left my office and headed to the car. I had said goodbye to Miss Mary in my heart many, many times as Alzheimer's gained ground. I hoped she felt free to leave us. As I drove, sunshine poured through clouds. "Thanks, Mama."

I parked and headed to the second floor, to her familiar room filled with pictures of grandchildren. I sat on the edge of her bed, my hand on her thin shoulder. She took labored breaths and opened her eyes. My sister said, "She waited." I said one last, "I love you, Mama," and within moments, her spirit was released from her diminished body and from the cruel tyrant Alzheimer's control. Her energy could not be destroyed. I said a final, "Amen" to a remarkable life.

Later, as I left Lakewood Manor and drove home past the cemetery where my mother would be joining my father, I thought about the Bon Secours Catholic hospice nurse. She had been by the bedside of hundreds of people at the end of life. She observed that people want to know three things when they are dying. I expected her to reply like a TV game-show host: so which will it be, 1) heaven, 2) hell or 3) purgatory? But the hospice nurse's response was far better: 1) did you give and receive love? 2) did you use your gifts? 3) did you make a difference? By all accounts, Mary Compton McMullin lived a full and remarkable life.

10:48 a.m.
January 24, 2013

16
Way-Enough

How much of life turns on a whisper, such as "I love you" or "Good bye?" My mother lied quietly in a nursing bed and exhaled for the last time with her life force leaving her body in a hushed whisper. A quiet passing with no need for words or loud sounds. As she was taking her last breath and leaving us, the nurse in a white uniform was entering the room.

After the moment your mother dies and leaves you alone for the first time, do you know what you do next? Fill out a form. The mystery of death is immediately followed by filling out a form in blue or black ink. The nurse on duty rolled down the white sheet covering my mother's still body and rolled up her pink pajama top to inspect her stomach to ensure that there was no movement, no more breathing. The facts were in: no vital signs.

"What time was Miss Mary's last breath, Mr. McMullin?"

"10:48 a.m."

"Thank you."

"Could you confirm her full legal name and date of birth?"

"Mary Compton McMullin."

"January 22, 1929."

"Do you know her social security number?" "Yes."

As my sister got her coat and walked out of the room, a second nurse was entering the room. Nurse #2 politely informed me, "Mr. McMullin, we need to collect your mother's jewelry and give it to you. Do you know where she kept it?"

"The jewelry box is in the top drawer of the dresser."

Her hands lifted the familiar cedar box with the silver plaque on the lid, a prize won at a golf tournament some 50 years ago. The dresser was made from Walnut trees on my grandfather James McMullin's farm. The wedding ring was given to her by my father, the opal ring from Aunt Betty and the beads from Aunt Clara. Time and space were spinning around me, as though I was the one with dementia-related vertigo. I reached for a chair, balanced and sat down.

"Thank you, Mr. McMullin. Would you like to take off her ring or would you like me to?"

"If you could, please." All jewelry was collected, put in the cedar box and handed to me. Next, her dementia-friendly wallet was passed my way. "Are there other valuables in the room, Mr. McMullin?"

"They would be in the top dresser drawer, next to her stash of chocolates."

Time for another form. I signed with a blue ink pen documenting that I had received my mother's valuables with the two nurses serving as witnesses. I chuckled at the process and could hear Miss Mary now, "I don't do money." In her lifetime, money held little value for Miss Mary and definitely not now.

The nurses were busy explaining practical next steps. Their words were taking flight but none were coming in for a landing. I saw their lips moving as someone handed me a piece of paper. I read the words at the top—my mother's room needed to be emptied of her belongings. I was being notified that if it was not emptied today, there were potential charges. Costs associated with her room could exceed $250 per day and these costs would be non-reimbursable from Medicare, Hospice, health insurance, long term care insurance. If it took me a week to clean it out, costs could exceed $2,000. In addition, there were potential fines.

My iPhone vibrated with my sister's text. She wanted the TV, in addition to the jewelry and dresser. Delivered to her house. She would not be returning to Lakewood. My brother would go ballistic over additional charges impacting his inheritance. And that could generate phone calls to lawyers and run up legal bills with a very high PIA factor. *Why was I thinking about lawyers and money?* My mind flashed back to the night when James and I bought and assembled the TV. Miss Mary wanted to see in high-definition clarity the golf ball during the US Open. I could hear her now, my mother with senile dementia. "Thank you, Darlin'. Can you imagine watching a tournament where you can't see the ball? An exercise in nonsense."

I texted my ever-compassionate and fair-minded sister, "All yours." I asked the kind social worker, "What is the last possible time for me to empty the room to avoid charges and fines?" Kelly replied, "No insurance company will pay past today. Could you do it before staff comes to work tomorrow morning?"

"Yes."

My mother may have exited to the Promised Land to laugh and dance with Bill in front of some celestial horn section, but I was still standing on Virginia red clay with plenty of red tape, corporate forms, insurance companies and lawyers. Right now, I wanted some time away from logistics. I called my wife and walked in a daze. My feet moved on their own accord and took me through the exit into the frigid January air. I looked through wet eyes and saw bare tree branches against vibrant blue sky. On autopilot, the SUV pulled out of Lakewood and took me home and pulled into our driveway. Marty and I hugged, both teary. I responded with all that remained to be said, "Make mine a double, Pussycat."

We headed to the neighborhood bar, ordered a drink and lunch. Cheers. And onto the next thing.

Every day has its work. But when the task in front of you is cleaning out your deceased mother's room, it is interesting to see who you instinctively call. With crisis as the great editor, I turned to Charlotte—Miss Mary's oldest grandchild—and without any hesitation she wanted to help. She didn't flinch or shed a tear when I explained we needed to pick out the clothes that her grandmother would wear to the grave. "I know what Grammy liked to wear, Popsicle." And she hugged me.

"What time?" was all DougE said.

So the team was assembled—Charlotte and DougE. No one could do any better.

That evening, Charlotte and I returned to Lakewood to begin the sorting. She was a pro now, having sorted Great Aunt Clara's jewelry and belongings. Grammy Mary's favorite things, photos, artwork by grandchildren, books were separated into three cardboard boxes of equal size: 1) Burke, 2) Keith, 3) Libby. We loaded trash bags with old makeup, bath soaps and underwear. I was the proud recipient of a lifetime supply of Kleenex tissue boxes. The final years of her life, Alzheimer's left her with a constant nasal drip. A Kleenex in the cuff of her blouse or sweater was as permanent as her opal ring.

Unbelievably, Miss Mary was down to a single rack of clothes in her closet. In a flash, Charlotte reached for her grandmother's favorite silk blouse and cornflower blue jacket. She loaded up a bag with shoes and other articles that might be needed. The outfit laid on the bed looked exactly like Miss Mary, but no one would ever see it other than me and Charlotte. My mom's directions were clear—no open casket.

We packed a box with other clothes to be donated to charity. We divided holiday decorations—wreaths for every season, Christmas tree, lights, pumpkins, valentines. When we got home, Char immediately hung the red heart wreath on the front door, shimmering in the light.

"Dad, what do you want to do with Grammy's canister of buttons?" My mother had carefully saved every button she had ever found and had hundreds available just in case she needed a replacement.

"No clue. Put it in my box for now."

"Why? Mom doesn't sew."

"At this moment, I'm not fully prepared to throw out an 85 year collection of buttons."

Char pretended to weigh the canister in her right hand. "Mmmmm, feels more like 75 years." The smart-ass gene remained with us.

"What about the Cribbage board and Backgammon game?"

"Divide the games between the boxes." Charlotte picked up velvet rectangular boxes with gold trim. Each held a matching set of playing cards with Audubon-like bird images that were used at countless Ladies' Bridge Luncheons. All I could hear in my mind was, *"Sugar, how about a quick hand of Gin Rummy?"*

A few things remained in the room unpacked. "Dad, what do you want to do with the lamp?"

"All to Aunt Libby. She can have it or give it to Burke or Goodwill. I'm done with stuff."

I texted Doug. We would meet at Starbucks at 5:45 a.m. the next morning and move the boxes and furniture by 6:30 a.m. with special delivery to Libby before 7:00 a.m. The room would be empty and broom clean before the facility staff started showing-up at Lakewood. I kept repeating, "Thanks, man." Doug replied, "You can stop thanking me now." But I knew with Miss Mary and Great Aunt Clara both gone, there was no one left to say "thank you" for extending a hand to help. Other than helping and thanking, what else mattered? Doug had a question of his own. "How come you don't fear getting Oldzheimerz?"

"I've always known Oldzheimerz. It is a given for me, and I assume that either Marty or I or both of us will likely die of it. In the words of Miss Mary, 'Let's focus on today and not borrow from tomorrow's trouble.'"

Once this morning's chores were done, I went by the cemetery where my father was buried. The director had pulled a file labeled "Mary C. McMullin." The file's paperwork was in perfect order. Unbelievably, Miss Mary had done it herself after being diagnosed with Alzheimer's dementia. Cemetery plot reserved. Head stone ordered, engraved and waiting on the date of death. All prepaid, with a Valpak discount coupon attached with a paperclip. I had no clue that cemeteries ran specials on dying. All that remained to do was for me to sign a stack of documents—so many forms of death.

My experience was the same at Woody Funeral Home. She had already met with them and pre-ordered her own casket and recorded her wishes—no open casket. She chose for herself exactly what had been selected for Aunt Clara. In her file was a piece of stationary with the names of hymns she liked. She had drafted the outline for an obituary with key accomplishments and dates. Miss Mary was hoping to rest in peace without troubling her children or causing arguments over her funeral arrangements or spending far too much money on emotional purchases. Her thoughtful and frugal spirit lived on.

At Woody's, I filled out a document that notified the Commonwealth of Virginia about her death. That one government form launched a fleet of ships. The Kayak Method went into steady gear to finalize her estate:

- Death certificates ordered
- Pensions terminated for both Mary and Bill
- Health insurance terminated
- Dental insurance terminated
- Pharmacy program terminated
- Lakewood final billing
- Long-term Care Insurance terminated
- Social Security notified
- Medicare notified
- Joint checking accounts closed
- Life insurance policies notified
- Final accounting completed with her lawyer
- Tax information to accountant
- Investment advisor contacted for distribution of accounts to beneficiaries
- Probate court contacted to schedule meeting to formalize executor

Then during a meeting at the office, my iPhone vibrated and my sister's name appeared on the screen. It was highly unusual for her to call, and I stepped outside the conference room to talk with her. There was a reason for the interruption. Her purpose was clear—had I rewritten our mother's will to benefit me and coerced her to sign it? She needed to know.

Way-enough was all I heard in my mind, the command to stop rowing when the race is finished. The moment in time had come for me to put the oar down. Miss Mary had already showed me how to resign as executor with Great Aunt Clara's estate. I called Paul Izzo, filled out the resignation form and hired Paul to represent me and my wife. With the resignation form officially notarized and stamped, I gave it to Paul and gave the control of my mother's money to Libby and Burke. My job as caregiver was done.

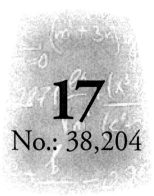

17
No.: 38,204

Pure and true religion before God the Father is this:
to care for orphans and widows in their misfortune...

James 1:27

I remember my feet sinking deep in the white powder sand and my heels making a squeaking sound as I trudged up the familiar dune, laughing with my brother, sister and cousin Betsy. I was probably eleven years old. Once I reached the top, out of breath, I could see the white beaches and dark green surf of the Atlantic rolling for miles to the north and south. Sea oats scratched my sunburned legs as I ran down the well-worn path toward the waves. The only human in sight was a white-bearded salty fisherman, standing knee deep in the surf near an abandoned and rusted-out boiler—the remains of a long-ago shipwreck.

Betsy and I ran and dove into the cold water, clothes and all, jumping over the smaller swells and body surfing the larger waves back to shore. In early summer, the air was far warmer than the seawater. For unmeasured time, we swam and joked and enjoyed the surf under an expanse of June blue sky.

In the 1960s and 70s, the North End of Virginia Beach was a beautiful deserted stretch of beach adjoining Fort Story Army Base, its own uninhabited waterfront used occasionally by the Army for amphibious-training purposes. These amphibians resembled a small battle ship encased in steel and jacked-up on tractor wheels for use on land or sea, like something out of a Mad Max movie. Silver rivets covered amphibians, along with tatted images of sharks teeth or Portuguese man-o'war. They spewed black diesel smoke as they ground their way from land directly into the ocean for mock battle. Dark green helicopters circled and made their whap-whap-whap birdcalls. The sea by Fort Story led to the mouth of the Chesapeake Bay, a hyperactive seaport with tankers and cargo ships, one after another, sailing in and out. My father, the Navy man, loved to surf fish and reliably carried his binocs with him, so we could watch the ships coming and going with our dreams on board.

This strip of abandoned Virginia Beach was steeped in history, and my father had read many books on the subject. Every summer we walked to the Cape Henry Light House, the first lighthouse built by the U.S. Government under the direction of President George Washington. We climbed the 191 steps to the beacon on top. Dripping in sweat and standing on the observation platform encased in glass, we had a perfect view of the coast line and "First Landing Beach." This was the place where, in 1607, Captain Christopher Newport came ashore and established Virginia in hope of a better life. When he landed in search of a new port, his team was seasick, hungry and completely out of beer. Close by, he established the first English settlement, called Jamestowne, on the banks of the James River. For my father, the lighthouse was an engineering marvel and climbing the centuries-old circular staircase was a fascinating voyage through time. I don't think he cared much about the sweat rolling off his face or ours as he pointed to where Revolutionary War battles had been fought at sea, right where we fished and surfed.

When I was growing up, enormous beach mansions for multiple families had not yet been invented with their wall-to-wall carpet, climate controlled air-conditioning and flat screen TVs. Our beach house at 108 89th Street was far more humble—more akin to camping. Miss Mary's best friend, Betty, told me that when she was a girl, the house was actually a store located about fifteen blocks away, where Fort Story is now. When the Army Base was built, the store was relocated to the last civilian street—89th Street. It was nothing more than a one-story house covered in grey shingles that had survived countless hurricanes and storms. A screened porch ran the width of the front of the house, and a second screened porch with a picnic table off the back served as our mess hall.

The outdoor shower stood ready under the back kitchen window, and in life, I was never once allowed to take a bath inside the house. Standing on a slippery wood palate claimed from a construction site, I welcomed the cool water from the rust-coated showerhead against my sunburned skin. I was required to wash the sand off all body parts with a bar of white Ivory soap and gold No More Tears shampoo before coming inside for dinner.

Scents are described as the strongest memory trigger, and I remember the smell of gardenias on the back steps of the house. An ancient bush with dark green glossy leaves seemed perennially in blooms, so perfectly formed they looked as if they were "Made in China" of white plastic. "Intoxicating" was Miss Mary's single-word response to the fragrance as she went up the concrete steps.

The house's wood floors were as worn as a ship's main deck. Generations of bare feet covered in beach sand had worn smooth the heart pine floors to shabby chic, long before anyone knew what that phrase meant. Electric fans circulated air through the house and hummed all summer. Floor to ceiling book shelves lining the large family room were haphazardly chock full of books, games and specimens of starfish, conch shells and horseshoe crabs. Whatever you found on those shelves was exactly how you could entertain yourself that summer. A rainy day at the beach is probably the only reason I ever learned to read or play Cribbage, my score pegged on a scrimshaw board crafted out of whalebone.

Unbelievable in today's world, there was no grocery store near our house on 89th Street. "Carry in, carry out" was the motto, and you ate what you brought with you from the suburbs. Miss Mary would cook a turkey and country ham in Richmond, pack them in the blue Coleman cooler and carry them with us to eat. A turkey sandwich with a slice of ripe tomato, sweet iceberg lettuce and a swipe of mayonnaise is still my idea of a perfect lunch. Every couple of days, the vegetable truck drove down 89th Street. Ringing an old ship's bell, a century-old waterman with an incomprehensible southern dialect sold Silver Queen corn, tomatoes, cantaloupe, peaches, limas and greens. We ordered fish and bushels of crabs from him, too. He had connections with the fishermen who docked at nearby Lynnhaven Inlet.

I remember my father finishing off one last beer before dinner, adding the empty can to the others in the bottom of the crab pot, covering the cans with water and heating it to a rolling boil. The pot was so large it covered two burners on the stovetop. He dropped blue crabs into this steaming hell—them pinching, scurrying, clawing and him showing no mercy. Inevitably, a large blue Jimmy or two would break free of the tongs and scuttle across the kitchen tile floor, pinchers opening and snapping closed. Kids hollered and jumped to safety on chairs; Bill laughed and nabbed them from behind with his bare hand. He chucked the ol' Jimmies into the pot, and with his other hand lowered the lid. The crab commotion was silenced. Shortly after, fire red crabs wearing a coat of orange Old Bay seasoning would hit the newspaper covered picnic table. And then the hard work would begin—cracking shells with pliers and using a nut pick to uncover sweet white crab meat, a delicacy of the mid-Atlantic.

We spent endless hours on the beach swimming, surfing on inflatable canvas rafts, fishing, building sandcastles, playing Frisbee, Kadima and beach golf. I can see Miss Mary sitting in her plaid beach chair about five inches above the sand. The former swimmer and lifeguard, behind Wayfarer sunglasses, kept one eye on the kids and one eye on her book. We debated the perennial topic of what time was really the BEST time at the beach: 1) early morning with the sunrise and a solitary fisherman, 2) afternoon with the clear blue sky and sun overhead, 3) 5:00 as the tide and cool air roll in, 4) evening as the sun sets with water color skies, or 5) nighttime with infinite stars and the moon reflecting on waves.

The winning answer was often option 3) 5:00 cocktail hour. I remember one of those evenings, my parents with a drink carried safely in a mason jar, smoking a cigarette and enjoying the ocean view. With the rhythm of the incoming waves, I heard Miss Mary observe, "When I look out over the ocean, I know in my heart that God is in heaven watching over his children, and love reigns supreme in our crazy world."

Like an attentive shepherd, she, too, was right there in her beach chair watching over her flock. A crazy world it is, full of the unexpected. Including for Mary and Bill, watching over three children they adopted as babies and raised as their own. My siblings and I were adopted—rescued—by Bill and Mary. This model couple of America's Greatest Generation—the successful and funny World War II vet, his beautiful and brilliant bride, the paid-for house, the golf and bridge champions—they were successful by any measuring stick. Miss Mary had achieved the American Dream in one generation, all except for having children.

After more than ten years of trying unsuccessfully to have a baby, including surgical procedures, in a prayerful moment they decided to adopt—not just one, not two, but three unwanted babies. And Miss Mary, the consummate school teacher, went about raising and educating her brood of strays just as she did the random students whose names turned up in her roll book each September. She knew how to teach anyone. A defining moment in her life, God answered her prayer in this crazy world. And as she said in her serene southern accent, "You are the child God intended me to raise." She believed it in her heart. And so would anyone, including me.

My buddy, DougE, and I were prone to joking that he was raised a "Trailer Park Bastard" with a young mother, and I was born a "Classic Bastard" to a young mother. His teenage mother brought him home from the hospital to raise in a rented trailer; mine gave me up for adoption. Neither one was an easy choice in the 1960s for a young woman, knocked up and carrying an unplanned baby. Whether or not the direct result of beer, bourbon and bad choices in the back seat, life can begin in a random moment of passion in this crazy world.

As the story goes, my birthmother and father were college students at University of Richmond while Miss Mary taught there. In the cryptic county paperwork, a social worker described my sperm-donor as "very good looking... a playboy type with little ambition," a completely out-of-bounds, yet hilarious, editorial comment for a social worker to record about my birth father's personality. I'm fond of the image in my mind's eye of him sitting in Miss Mary's classroom, eyes rolling and thinking about seeing his girlfriend as Miss Mary expertly solved problems on the blackboard. (Now let's see, if Parent A was replaced with the variable Parent B, what would happen to Baby C?) I also like to imagine Bill's strong arm holding me as a tiny baby and what he might say about the entire situation with the college playboy: "That won't do." The strong hand of Bill, the sure hand of Mary and the invisible hand of God all guided this lost baby sheep.

The circumference of my life experience could be measured in about a two-mile radius. From conception with unnamed University of Richmond college co-eds, to being born and recorded as baby no.: 38,204 in The Book of Life, to a happy childhood with Mary and Bill, to preschool through grade twelve, to middle age with my own wife and kids, I haven't lived much farther than these two miles. I've always felt the details of my life story are both random and hilarious. There is the love of God, there is the grace of God, and clearly there is the humor of God.

I'm sure for my birthmother, however, her situation in 1965 was not a laughing matter. From a family of doctors, nurses and Episcopal ministers, being unmarried and pregnant was, I feel sure, neither her plan nor her parents'. In the time before Roe v. Wade, a quiet abortion would not have been easy, and her boyfriend was not the marrying kind. Dating and sex with him may have been fun in the spring, but as the weather turned cold, the situation was not so funny. As life would have it, she more than likely went into labor to birth this love child on Valentine's Day, with Bill's golf buddy by her side as the attending physician who delivered me.

While kayaking and fishing and drinking beer with Doug, he has pointed out to me that in my heart I am a religious person. For me, the defining moment in my life was a moment of God's grace. I believe that the God of the universe intervened in my life and guided Mary and Bill to adopt me when I was an unwanted and one hundred percent dependent newborn. Miss Mary outstretched her hand, took me in, held me close and raised me as her own.

And when she was lost to Alzheimer's dementia and was in the process of becoming completely dependent, I, in turn, reached out my hand to help her. I was not born her son; loving care made me her son. Life isn't about being perfect or developing a foolproof plan. Getting knocked-up by a handsome playboy isn't about true love or a perfect relationship. Contracting Alzheimer's disease and slowly dying one brain cell at a time is not about perfect health or a timely death. As Miss Mary assessed—we will make the best of a bad situation. The best you can do is extend your hand to help those in need as best you can, today. And if you choose not to reach out, no one else may help either. And no one may help you one day in your darkest hour of greatest need.

Like Uncle Sol recruiting a teacher and reformer from Wellesley College for the pioneer settlement school in the mountains of Kentucky, we all have the power to make a difference far beyond our imagination and our generation. After all, I am Uncle Sol's great-great-great grandson grafted in the family tree by adoption, telling the story of his great-great granddaughter's remarkable life. No one could have imagined this story. After Miss Mary's funeral, I received countless letters and cards from people I had never met. Not one mentioned her noteworthy accomplishments. But everyone remembered how she made them feel special and loved. Emotional memory is strongest. The most powerful lesson Miss Mary taught me came through her death by Alzheimer's dementia—love reigns supreme in our crazy world.

Amen

The 3 Ds: Dementia, Alzheimer's Disease, Delirium

Compiled from Subject Matter Experts at Johns Hopkins
University School of Medicine

Dementia

Alzheimer's disease is the most common type of dementia. Worldwide, it accounts for 60-80% of all reported cases of dementia. Dementia refers to a significant intellectual decline that persists over time and affects several areas of cognition or thinking. The condition is often not diagnosed until months or even years after its onset. Memory loss is a universal feature of dementia, but other functions are impaired, such as abstract thinking and language.

After Alzheimer's disease, the most common cause of significant memory loss is Vascular Dementia—a disorder often resulting from a series of tiny strokes that destroy brain cells. Other types of dementia include Dementia with Lewy Bodies, Frontotemporal Dementia and Huntington's Disease.

Alzheimer's Disease

A person in the United States develops Alzheimer's disease every 68 seconds. The progressive brain disorder is characterized by a gradual deterioration of mental faculties caused by a loss of nerve cells and the connections between them. Alzheimer's is often accompanied by changes in behavior and personality. People who are 65 and older survive an average of four to eight years after the initial diagnosis.

The human brain is extremely complex with 86 billion nerve cells, and there is no certainty that scientists will fully understand its working anytime soon—even though the brain is responsible for such significant actions as memory, behavior and consciousness. Science has not yet pinpointed the true cause of Alzheimer's. Traditional theories are based on two factors: 1) neurofibrillary tangles and 2) amyloid plaques.

- **Tangles** are composed mostly of a protein called tau. These hairlike threads are what remain after a neuron's internal support structure collapses. In healthy nerve cells, these threads function like train tracks to carry nutrients from one destination to another. In Alzheimer's, the protein threads becomes hopelessly twisted and useless.
- **Plaques** are a mixture of abnormal proteins and cell fragments that form in the tissue between nerve cells. Amyloid plaques are gooey and become toxic in areas of the brain responsible for memory, learning and planning. As nerve cell destruction spreads, more of the brain is impacted, especially in the cerebral cortex, which is responsible for reasoning and language. As Alzheimer's disease progresses, large areas of nerve cells die, brain sections atrophy and the whole brain shrinks in size.

Delirium

Delirium and dementia can coexist in one patient, but they are not the same thing. Dementia comes on gradually and is a permanent condition. Delirium is an abrupt change that comes on suddenly and is short-lived, lasting anywhere from hours to days. When a person becomes delirious, it means he or she is confused or disoriented and has difficulty thinking clearly and focusing. People with delirium may not remember events and often misperceive and misinterpret their surroundings—or may not be aware of them. Delirium affects nearly one-third of patients over the age of 65 admitted to hospitals and is most common with patients in the intensive care unit (ICU).

References

Karin J. Neufeld, M.D., M.P.H. "Recognizing and Treating Delirium." *Memory Disorders Bulletin*, Fall 2014, Johns Hopkins Medicine, 28–40.

Peter V. Rabins, M.D., M.P.H. "introductory article to Memory Disorders Bulletin." *Memory Disorders Bulletin*, Winter 2014, Johns Hopkins Medicine, 1–14.

Peter V. Rabins, M.D., M.P.H. "Looking Ahead." *Memory Disorders Bulletin,* Spring 2014, Johns Hopkins Medicine, 3–24.

Peter V. Rabins, M.D., M.P.H. "The Biology of Memory." *Memory White Paper*, 2014, John Hopkins Medicine, 1–4.

Peter V. Rabins, M.D., M.P.H. "Irreversible Dementias" and "Alzheimer's Disease." *Memory White Paper*, 2014, John Hopkins Medicine, 33–65.

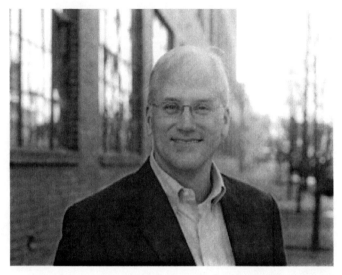
Photo courtesy of Scott Elmquist.

J. Keith McMullin has led health care program development, marketing and sales for more than 20 years in local and national markets. A graduate of the University of Virginia, he currently leads medical fundraising for Bon Secours St. Mary's Hospital, homecare and hospice in Richmond, Virginia. He learned first-hand how to be successful amidst constant changes and uncertainty in the health care industry through his second full-time job—caregiving for his mom with Alzheimer's disease. *Missing Mary* is his first book. He can be reached at his website, www.missingmary.com.

.